MY BAGS WERE ALWAYS PACKED

(A Mother's Journey Through Her Son's Cancer Treatment And Remission)

Elizabeth F. Szewczyk

Copyright © 2006 by Elizabeth F. Szewczyk

All rights reserved. No part of this book shall be reproduced or transmitted in any form or by any means, electronic, mechanical, magnetic, photographic including photocopying, recording or by any information storage and retrieval system, without prior written permission of the publisher. No patent liability is assumed with respect to the use of the information contained herein. Although every precaution has been taken in the preparation of this book, the publisher and author assume no responsibility for errors or omissions. Neither is any liability assumed for damages resulting from the use of the information contained herein.

ISBN 0-7414-3022-3

Published by:

INFINITY
PUBLISHING.COM

1094 New DeHaven Street, Suite 100
West Conshohocken, PA 19428-2713
Info@buybooksontheweb.com
www.buybooksontheweb.com
Toll-free (877) BUY BOOK
Local Phone (610) 941-9999
Fax (610) 941-9959

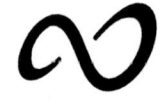

Printed in the United States of America
Printed on Recycled Paper
Published January 2006

There are so many people who have helped me
to bring this book to publication.

To John S. for encouraging me in his Memoirs class—thanks for the honesty and the inspiration.

To Jack, Laura, Rosemary, Mike, Deirdre, Bill, Rick, Seanna—I couldn't ask for more wonderful brothers and sisters. You always helped me believe.

To Elaine—We've been friends for over thirty years and I thank God for you every day. The early readings at breakfast always made me laugh.

To JoAnn—My prayer partner. We're always praying for our children together. Since that first day of Dan and Mike's Kindergarten class, you have been here for me.

Cathy and Steve—How on earth did you remember to send Dan a card every week? We are so grateful to be part of your family.

To Father K. and Father Bill—Every prayer, every blessing gave me strength to go on.

To Joyce C.—Dan was blessed with your teaching methods in second grade and blessed again with your prayers and holy medals. Thank you.

To Cioci Theresa and Uncle Rudy—You were always positive, always loving.

To Mom and Dad S.—You have my love and heart always.

To Dad F.—Great moments, great hope, great love, come from you.

Thank you all for caring, for loving, for being there.

To Mom and Brenda—Your gift of life sustains us all.

To Ryan and Tom R.—You are loved like sons.

Dear Allison, Tommy, Jessica and Dan—My four miracles.

And to Tom, who continues to love me after all these years in spite of myself. You are my soul mate, my deepest joy. I couldn't have written this without your inspiration.

The author happily shares equal portions of the sale of this book with children's cancer research and the Make-A-Wish Foundation® of Connecticut.

Dedication

For Dan

"Before you were born I knew you.
I have carved your name in the palm
of My hand."

Isaiah 49

Introduction

Having a child with a life threatening illness and going through the diagnosis and treatment is like no other pain I've known. When it became clear that Daniel had cancer, my life changed forever. I joined the mothers who live day-by-day hoping and praying that their child would get well. I witnessed mothers who cried inconsolably when their prayers weren't answered the way they'd hoped. I rejoiced with mothers whose children finished treatment and were able to rejoin a life of "new normal." There were mothers who relied on their faith in God to carry them through each crisis and mothers who denied any existence of God. What each of these women had in common with me was that we loved our children. We loved their life. We held them in our arms when they were babies and held them again as they fought for life. And any of us would gladly have changed places with them if it meant they would be spared the hurt cancer causes.

Daniel is one of the survivors. He went through his treatment and continues to be strong and healthy. He is an inspiration of triumph in spite of obstacles and an example of how I'd like to live the rest of my life. He doesn't remember everything that happened during his treatment but I often remind him how brave he was and continues to be.

This book is the final chapter of a journal I kept when Dan was diagnosed and treated. When he was sick there were so many parents who contacted our family to let us know we weren't alone. Hopefully, this book will let other parents know that they are not alone during this terrible time. There are thousands of parents who pray for you and your child daily. We pray for miracles and I know they happen. Dan is a miracle. This is our story.

Daniel's story takes place at the beginning of springtime, 2001. Daniel is a lively, loving boy with a great sense of humor. He whistles as he passes by and sings in the shower. He always has a joke at the dinner table. Dan has dark chestnut brown hair that falls straight on his forehead and huge brown eyes. His skin is an olive shade; even in the winter he looks as though he is tan. He has an athletic build from years of playing soccer and weight training. He is to all who see him, "the picture of health." In April of 2001, I noticed a bump on Daniel's right leg, toward the outside where the tendon bends the kneecap. He didn't say it hurt but it was noticeably there. I thought that it was a bug bite or a soccer injury. Either way, I wasn't concerned. Dan had had his share of bumps and bruises over the years from soccer. I cast this bump off as another "battle wound" from an intense game.

Spring always brings forth busyness in the Szewczyk's extra-curricular schedule. With a large extended family, our weekends are filled with First Communions, graduations, soccer games and chorus concerts. Meals are eaten on the run as we head toward another event. So I told myself that Daniel's lump would go away—it was nothing of consequence. Our lives were too hectic to be concerned over something that seemed to be trite.

Spring gave way to summer. I finished teaching for the year and my husband Tom and I were celebrating our twenty-fifth wedding anniversary. We were planning a cruise to Bermuda at the beginning of July. We had cruised to Bermuda three years before and were enchanted with the people, the flora and the fauna. Tom loved scouting the pristine beaches for unusual shells. He would weave in and out of coves, always finding something new to add to his beach collection at home. The crystal blue water in Bermuda mirrored the sea life beneath the foaming waves and low tide brought an abundance of treasures. While Tom walked along the waters I would sit under an umbrella, reading the latest mystery book "hot off the presses." Without the frantic pace of home, Bermuda became our haven.

June came and soccer season was almost over. Our oldest daughter, Allison, had just completed a degree in English from Framingham State College. She and her boyfriend Ryan, announced their engagement shortly before graduation. We were thrilled that Ryan would be joining our family. Tommy, our oldest son, was settling into his own apartment, working full time and taking classes at a community college. He was gaining responsibility and growing into a fine man. Jessica, our youngest daughter, was anxiously looking forward to attending chorus camp in Ohio. Jessica would be heading into her senior year of high school and music was a strong part of her life. Daniel was ready to begin high school in September. Tom and I were proud of the goals our children had set. We felt pleased to be heading into a new realm of parenthood. Our children were leaving familiar surroundings and were ready to embark on a new journey of independence. With this newfound freedom, Tom and I often enjoyed quiet dinners; evenings at the movies or time spent at home reading. Our life seemed somewhat settled and very happy.

Meanwhile, Daniel's lump had noticeably grown. It was about the size of a marble, perfectly round and most alarming of all, painless. Painless to the touch, painless when trying to move it, painless when squeezing it. I found this unsettling because I had read so many articles on cancer detection. I knew that a lump that continued to grow without movement and pain signaled cause for alarm.

I have a theory that there is a gift women receive when they become mothers. It is an intuition, a bonding of sorts that joins the mother to the child in a protective, nurturing manner. I believe the bond continues throughout the child's life. This is the only way I can explain how I knew something was wrong with Dan; that the growth was not something temporary but that it had reached the point of concern.

I made an appointment with Dr. Warren, our family doctor, to have the lump examined. Like most appointments that involved our sons, I asked Tom to take Dan to the doctor.

"I think the lump needs to be checked. I don't think it's a bug bite. It's hard and immobile. It doesn't hurt when I try to squeeze it or flatten when I push down on it. Would you tell Dr. Warren I've noticed it for three months? Wouldn't a bug bite have gone away by now?"

Tom agreed it needed to be looked at. After a soccer game in June, off he went with Dan to see Dr. Warren. Dr. Warren had taken care of Dan since he was born. He had a kind, caring manner with a great sense of humor. He could calm even the most frenzied parent. During the children's baby years, I was often that parent. Over the years I had developed a great respect for him.

Dr. Warren assured Tom and Dan that there was no cause for alarm. In fact, he thought the lump was probably a cyst or scar tissue from a soccer injury. But to be on the safe side, he recommended the lump be removed and referred Dan to a surgeon.

"Can it wait until after soccer season?" Dan asked.

"Sure. There's no hurry to take it out." Dr. Warren replied. "Just make sure you have the surgeon look at it when the season is over."

So we waited. I looked at it often.

"Are you sure it doesn't hurt?"

"I'm sure, mom. It doesn't feel like anything."

I should have been glad that this thing was painless each time I subjected Dan to the squeezing and poking. But instinctively my heart would skip a beat or two each time he told me it didn't hurt.

"What if I push down on it?"

"No, mom."

"How about if I squeeze it a bit?"

"Nothing, mom. It doesn't feel like anything."

My heart sank. How on earth would I cope if this thing were more than a soccer injury? I immediately put the thoughts of sickness and fear out of my mind. We made an appointment at the end of June with Dr. McDonald, a well-known surgeon.

The day before the appointment we celebrated Dan's fourteenth birthday with presents, a fancy dinner, and his favorite chocolate cake. Tom and I went overboard with presents, buying him more than we had intended. Shirts and shorts, soccer equipment, video games, cd's and movies. We showered him with everything on his list. I watched Dan open his gifts and devour chocolate cake, thanking God for his life, his health and praying that both would continue.

"You've blessed us with thirteen years to love him, Lord." I prayed. "Thank you for these years. Please watch over him for thirteen more."

After his cake and presents, Dan asked to go to his friend Michael's house. Michael had been his best buddy since kindergarten, when he rescued a nervous Dan from trying to escape his new classroom. Dan and Mike grew up together, each year becoming more and more like brothers than friends. Still, I hesitated.

"Don't you want to hang around here a while longer? Maybe you could play some of your new games?"

"Nah." He answered. "I'll just take them to Mike's. We'll probably go swimming too."

"Okay." I relented. "Take a towel so that Mrs. Swift doesn't have to give you one and be home at ten o'clock."

It was the last time Dan would swim that summer.

~~~~~~~~~~~~~~~~~~~

In the morning, Tom and I accompanied Dan to the doctor's office. Dr. McDonald had performed several operations on me and other members in my extended family. He had a wonderful, warm bedside manner, was an outstanding surgeon technically and was well respected in the town community.

"It looks like a cyst or some type of benign growth, nothing of alarm," said the doctor. "Still, it should be removed." He measured the lump and recommended hospital day surgery rather than an office removal. He wasn't quite sure how deep the growth was and whether blood vessels were involved. Tom and I mentioned we were scheduled to leave on July seventh for a cruise to Bermuda.

"It's our twenty-fifth wedding anniversary. We had plans to go to Bermuda. But if Dan's surgery can't be performed before we go, we'll cancel our trip."

"No, no," Dr. McDonald assured us. "Let me call the hospital right now. They can usually fit these surgeries in right away. Of course he'll need to stay off his leg until the stitches are removed."

Dr. McDonald immediately called the hospital, pulled a few strings and arranged for surgery on July fifth.

"Who will be with Dan after the surgery?" he asked.

Tom and I told him Dan would recuperate at his grandparent's house while we went on the cruise. Dr. McDonald scheduled a post-op appointment for the following Friday when Dan would have his stitches removed. I was perfectly agreeable to this arrangement.

July fifth came. Dan was scheduled for a nine-thirty morning procedure that would not require general anesthesia. He seemed so grown-up walking into the hospital, checking himself in with the Admission's nurse, having his blood drawn and getting an IV put into his arm. I tried to "mother" him by rubbing his shoulders and back but he wanted no part of it.

"Mom, I'm ok. Stop, please."

Little did I know there would be plenty of time for mothering.

Forty-five minutes after he walked into the operating room the surgery was finished. Dr. McDonald met us in the waiting room.

"It was a solid tumor," he said, shaking his head in disbelief. There was a sharp tone in his voice. He seemed astonished.

"But it looked completely benign," he added, as if trying to convince himself and us that the trauma would end here. We thanked him for his time and expertise as we were escorted to the recovery room to see Dan.

There he was, wrapped in a white and blue hospital gown, three sizes too large.

"Can you believe the size of my bandage? All this gauze for that little bump!"

We nodded. Half of his kneecap was covered with bandage. Dan continued,

"Nothing hurt. I couldn't even believe when it was over. Can we go home now?"

The Novocain hadn't worn off and he was comfortable enough to be anxious to leave this confining area. Dr. McDonald walked in to discharge him.

"Go on your cruise. He's going to be just fine."

Tom and I heaved a sigh of relief. Our son was going to be fine and we were going to set sail for Bermuda in two days! Dan's recuperation for the week at his Bobcie and Dzadzie's was a comfortable feeling. Bobcie would insist he stay off his leg, making him French toast breakfasts with all the chocolate milk he could drink. She would fluff his pillows, change the movies in the VCR and fuss over him all week. Dzadzie would come home after work and they'd play cards or board games. After a few hours Dzadzie would go out for ice cream sundaes and more movies. In other words, Dan's week would be "Heaven." He'd rest and be spoiled. On Friday, Bobcie would bring him to Dr. McDonald where his stitches would be removed. Then Tommy would take him home on Friday night so Dan could settle in at home before our return. We would be home on Saturday.

~~~~~~~~~~~~~~~~~~~~~~~~~~~~~~~

Taking a cruise is the ultimate way to indulge your fantasies. From preparing meals to seeing that your bed is turned down at nighttime, the crew meets every need. It is a paradise on water and Tom and I treated it as such. We ate salmon and filet, drank wine spritzers by poolside and slept to the ocean's rocking as the ship cruised on the sea.

We both reflected on the joy of raising four wonderful children. We laughed about their desire to live near or at home after warning us how they "couldn't wait to get out of the house." They were a close bunch, confiding in each other, happy for one another's triumphs. Life was good. I thought of the lazy, carefree summer approaching, before Jessica's senior year and Dan's freshman year. It was going to be a time of relaxation, of not having to keep track of every move our children took. I thought of this as the greatest chapter in our lives, with a sense of freedom and new exploration. Little did I know my world as I knew it was about to end, to dissolve like a vapor on a cold winter's night. One single word would blow it away forever.

We called our children on Friday night to ask how they had fared during their first real week of independence.

"Everything is fine," Allison casually answered. "Danny? Oh he's good. He's sleeping over Mike's tonight. Yes, his stitches are out. What time should I pick you up from the bus station?"

Allison would be driving her new car and sounded excited for us to come home. Tommy took the phone to say hello, ask how the trip was and tell us he'd see us tomorrow. We didn't "chat" since this one call was exorbitantly expensive. There would be plenty of time to share our trip on Saturday night. On Sunday, Jessica would return from her week at chorus camp in Ohio. I had chaperoned the trip to Ohio two years before and knew it was a week packed with adventure. She would have stories to share, dancing and singing to perform for us. I couldn't wait to see my children now. This trip had been just long enough. Tom and I spent the final night of our cruise packing. How on earth would we carry all of these souvenirs off the ship? This seemed our greatest concern on that last night.

Cruises are magnificent until the day of disembarkment. Passengers are given colored tags the last evening and in the morning are herded into a large lounge until their color is announced over the loud speaker. Usually the wait is two or three hours. Tom and I passed the time reading, talking and drinking coffee, anxious to "get the show on the road." What little patience we have toward non-catastrophic events! Finally our color was called. We thanked the crew for their excellent service, disembarked and boarded a luxury bus headed for home. Another couple, our dinner partners each evening, boarded the same bus. They looked as tired and anxious as we did. This paradise was definitely over.

~~~~~~~~~~~~~~~~~~~~~~~~~~~

Three hours past our anticipated arrival, due to bus malfunctions and heavy traffic, we pulled into the Hartford bus terminal. We were exhausted! Dragging our bags, looking very much like irritable tourists, we spotted Allison in the parking lot. She waved and smiled.

"How was your trip?" she asked, hugging us tightly. She lingered in our arms a little longer than usual.

"Everything was great," we responded as we loaded our bags into the trunk. "Are Tommy and Dan home?"

"Everyone's home. Everyone's waiting to see you."

As she drove along the empty highway we told her about the cruise, the sights of Bermuda, the weather and the shopping. She listened quietly, nodding her head occasionally. I assumed her silence was due to our constant chatting and the fact that her attention was focused on the safety of her new car. I felt relaxed, content and delighted with life. Approaching home we asked Allison about the new job she had recently started and also how our three dogs had fared in our absence. We asked about Dan's leg.

"Did Bobcie take Dan to the doctor's yesterday?"

"Oh yes. He had his stitches removed. His leg healed fine. Tommy brought him home from Bobcies' yesterday afternoon."

In retrospect, I am overwhelmed by her brave composure as she carried on this conversation.

I have never known what a premonition really felt like until we pulled into our driveway that afternoon and I saw Bobcies' car parked in front of our home. Why would she be here at this hour? Danny had come home from her house yesterday after his doctor appointment. Unlike previous vacations, she hadn't looked after the dogs. Why would she be here now?

"Your mom's car is here, Tom," I stated in a concerned tone. "Do you think something's wrong with your father?"

Tom looked at me, shrugged his shoulders, and quickly headed up the driveway to our porch.

We walked into the unusually silent house where Bobcie, Tommy and Danny were sitting in the family room, looking worn and tired. A cold wave of unsettlement passed through me.

"Oh my God," I thought. "Someone has died."

I don't remember anyone asking how our trip was, although I'm sure they did. What I do remember is Tom's mother saying words that will be forever embedded in my mind.

"When Dr. McDonald got the pathology report, it showed that Danny has cancer. It's a type called Large T-cell Non-Hodgkin's Lymphoma. Dr. McDonald was shocked by the report; the operation never gave him a clue that it could be so serious." She stopped to compose her voice.

"He told me Dan would probably need some chemotherapy and maybe some radiation. He gave me a copy of the pathology report for you to read."

Tears ran from her eyes.

"He also said he'd call you on Monday and had already called the children's hospital to get Danny set up for treatment."

By this time, everyone in the room except me was crying, hugging Dan and hugging each other. Do you know what I did? I walked swiftly past this frenzy and into the quiet dining room. I looked through a weeks' worth of mail! I searched the mail for bills, letters, offers of charge cards at four percent. Spreading the letters over the surface of the carved oak table I completely detached myself from the situation—but only for this moment in time. Wails of sorrow and fear flowed through our home. I couldn't take part in this distress, not until my mind had registered the implications of that word: Cancer. Cancer. Dan has Cancer. My mind reeling in shock, knowing that nothing would ever be the same, I reached for a bit of normal, grasping at the routine in everyday life. I checked the mail.

When Dan became sick it stopped our world and all plans of the immediate future stopped with it. Nothing mattered but Dan's health. My mind focused on his future, his past and his life. Would he get married? Would he have children? Live to his senior year? What could have been done to prevent this? What could be done to cure this? I felt like a broken soul. As a mother I prayed to God to give me this tragedy rather than to Dan. I soon realized the tragedy belonged to us all; Dan was just the main component.

On Sunday morning Tom and I went to Mass. Sitting there, listening to the readings and homily, I looked around at the congregation. I wanted to stand up, say to these people I'd known for years,

"Listen to me! Our son Danny has cancer. He may never get life insurance, marry or even graduate from high school. And where are You now, God? I'd like to pull You from that cross and shake You for what You've allowed to happen to my son!"

Instead, for the first time since I was told his diagnosis, I cried. Huge, gasping sobs finally released from my body. I cried for Danny and the impending hurt I knew he'd suffer. I cried for our family, now disrupted by disease. I cried for Tom and myself and the agony parents experience when their child is very sick. My head throbbed, my body shook and my heart ached. I was oblivious to my surroundings. I was entwined within the rope of suffering. Laura H. leaned over the pew and asked if I was sick.

"No," I squeaked. "Danny has cancer."

"I'm so sorry. What can I do to help?" she whispered.

"I don't know, Laura. I can't believe this. I just can't believe this."

The last few words gutted from my throat, choking me. I wailed and couldn't catch my breath. Tom clasped my shoulder, squeezing me to his chest. Laura hugged Tom, said she was terribly sorry and left. The word "cancer" kept repeating in my head.

After Mass Tom walked into the vestibule and told Father K. that Danny would need some very strong prayers. With optimism he would retain throughout Danny's illness, Tom relayed Dan's diagnosis. Father K., who I'd known since I was seven years old, wrapped his arm around my shoulder, reminding me to have faith. I was still crying. The tears felt like a pelting rain on my cheeks. I imagined Mary, the mother of Jesus, watching her son suffer at His cross. I wondered how I could possibly be as strong.

As we waited for Monday, Tom remained positive. He read and re-read the pathology report and concluded that the cancer was caught early and Dan would be fine with treatment. I couldn't accept this as faithfully. I wanted Dan well now. I didn't want him to have pain or lose his hair or be anything but a normal fourteen-year-old boy. I wanted to turn back the clock, to watch Dan fuss over his hair and stomp his feet when soccer games were lost to another team. Life was so much easier then and I had taken the loveliness for granted. I kept asking Tom questions about the pathology report over and over. I so wanted it to be a mistake. I prayed for a mistake.

One of the hardest times during this weekend was telling our family members, especially Jessica, who had been away at camp. There was no time for her to relish the return to home. She sensed the disruption immediately and took the news very hard. Dan is her baby brother and she protects him as much as she teases him. I comforted her in a half-hearted way, too possessed by my own grief.

"Life is not fair, no matter how much you want it to be," I kept saying.

Our family called us throughout the day. My sisters Laura and Rosemary offered meals and company; my sisters-in law Deirdre and Seanna offered the same. My brothers Jack and Michael wanted to take Dan to a ballgame or movie. My father reassured me that this was only temporary; Dan would be well again. Tom's brothers called in the evening with words of hope and love across the miles. His parents came over with dessert, still stunned by the news. Tom's aunt and uncle, Cioci Theresa and Uncle Rudy, sat with us during coffee and relayed stories of people with cancer who were perfectly fine after treatment. I thanked them all for the love they gave. In the months that followed, I would thank them again and again.

Meanwhile, life moved on. Dan wanted to be with his friends and forget about tomorrow (we were headed for the hospital on Monday for a consultation.). I let him leave, mainly at his insistence. What I really wanted to do was tightly hold him to myself, protecting him forever. But knowing he needed to be with his friends to forget the moment, I let him go. After he'd left, I searched the Internet for information about Dan's disease. I found news of a ninety-percent cure rate with intense chemotherapy and side effects of mouth sores, anemia and blood transfusions. How could I subject my son to all of this for ninety percent? Then, catching my breath, I realized I would subject him to this for nine percent, just for the chance at a long, healthy life. But it was excruciating to think of Dan reacting to pain deliberately induced to create wellness. My head throbbed.

We passed the time until Monday mundanely watching television. I cried a lot. Tom sighed a lot. The cruise seemed years ago. Maybe tomorrow we would have more information and answers I thought. I closed my eyes and lay my head on the soft quilted couch. My life was forever changed. I was the mother of a cancer patient. Is that how we'd identify Dan? Was this his legacy? The tears fell again. I was engulfed in an overwhelming sense of grief for my healthy son who was now so sick.

Journal Entry:

Monday finally arrives—a beautiful day. It is hot, sunny and alive with the sweet sounds of summer. I listen to the birds chirping loudly in their nests lodged within our maple trees and wonder what they might be saying. Are they singing of life and the beauty it brings when their nests are filled with newborn babies? I move onto the open front porch attached to our white colonial home. It's a favorite summer ritual of mine to drink my first cup of morning coffee on this porch sitting in a rocking chair and watching the world go by. Today is different. I am restless from a fitful sleep and anxious about the hospital.

Dressing in silence I think about my youngest child. Dan came into this world with a bang, all ten pounds one ounce of him. Tom and I were prepared for his cesarean birth but were not prepared for me to be awake and alert, with Tom present in the delivery room. When the doctor delivered Daniel we were mesmerized. This perfect bundle with deep chocolate brown eyes and stubbly black hair looked at us as we grasped his tiny fingers in our hands. He was so beautiful. Like our other children before him, we fell in love with him immediately. The nurses swaddled him in soft downy blankets and put him gently on my chest. Tom and I were stunned once again at the miracle of life. So now, fourteen years later, as I prepared to take my "miracle" for cancer treatment, I relived that day.

Walking into the children's hospital we were greeted by smiling, upbeat nurses and receptionists, which I thought was very odd. I expected an environment of tears and sorrow, of feelings that were my own. I walked into the opposite. Dr. Hamilton came out to inspect us. He was young, younger than I imagined, with a wide smile, round glasses and an impish look on his face. His youth made me nervous. How much experience could he possibly have? He shook our hands after the introductions and quickly focused on Dan. He checked his scar and thought he felt two swollen lymph nodes behind his knee.

"How much worse can this get?" I wondered out loud.

The tears were on the surface of my eyes again. Then as Tom and I were ushered to the waiting room, Dr. Hamilton led Dan into the examining room. I thought of the brave boy who walked to the operating room two weeks before and I let the tears fall once more.

When Dr. Hamilton and Dan came into the waiting room thirty minutes later, Dr. Hamilton looked contemplative and older. He motioned for us to sit in the far corner of the room where we would have privacy. Dan joined us, wanting to hear everything that was going to happen.

"You have two options," he started. "One is a chemotherapy regimen that has a three day, two week off schedule. It requires hospital stay but that is mainly to give a constant dose of chemotherapy. Patients react well to this regimen with few side effects. After three days they go home until two weeks later. During their time home, they pretty much function as usual, resuming normal activities, even attending school. The cure rate of this protocol is seventy to eighty percent."

"What's the other option?" Tom asked, hesitant to hear about the horrific drugs he often had to order for his customers who were on chemotherapy.

Dr. Hamilton paused and held his breath for a slight second. His blue eyes narrowed as he spoke to us in a lower decibel.

"The other option requires a five day hospitalization. Two weeks between each treatment is crucial to allow the patient's blood levels to recover. The patient's reaction is more intense. Dan would be the first patient at this hospital to undergo this protocol. But the cure rate is ninety five percent."

Tom and I looked at each other, afraid of hearing the rest of the protocol.

"Patients may get mouth sores, severe anemia requiring transfusions and platelets, stomach ulcerations, heart defects and growth retardation." He lowered his head.

"Is that all?" I stammered.

"No," Dr. Hamilton paused. "Dan's staging calls for four rounds of treatment. I would suggest six rounds, but it's your decision."

The room became silent. I held Tom's hand a little tighter.

Dr. Hamilton asked, "Are there any questions?"

For the first time since Dan's diagnosis I thought clearly.

"How will we know that the treatment has worked?"

"Good question. We'll be fairly certain the cancer is gone if it doesn't reappear within two months after treatment has ended."

I mentally counted the months ahead. That meant January. It seemed a very long time until January. Then Dan spoke:

"Will I lose my hair?"

"Yes, Dan, you will," Dr. Hamilton replied softly. "I'm sorry."

I wondered how we could make this decision. Why had our lives suddenly become so complicated? I looked at Dan and thought of all the years he still had to live, to explore his life and everything it held for him. I thought of his character; he wasn't a quitter and had weathered difficult times before. In my mind I traveled to his birth and how Tom and I promised him the world. And then I knew what the decision had to be. We would give Dan the best chance to cure this disease. Tom looked into my eyes and I knew he felt the same.

And so it was decided. The second option and the first of six rounds would begin in one week, after a catheter was surgically implanted in Danny's chest to administer his chemotherapy as painlessly as possible.

~~~~~~~~~~~~~~~~~~~~

On July 19, 2001, Danny was scheduled to enter the hospital to have a catheter port placed under his left shoulder muscle. Unfortunately, this day was also Allison's twenty-second birthday. In our home, we celebrate birthdays in a big way. We put up signs all over the kitchen and dining room walls professing our love for the birthday person. We have a special breakfast with blueberry pancakes, French toast, fresh fruit and vegetarian sausages. Presents are usually given at this time along with a special cake. We sing "Happy Birthday" with a Pavarotti bravado, even giving an encore if requested. We began this tradition when the children were born because it worked so well with Tom's schedule. It's a time for our family to enjoy our life and love the birthday person with all our hearts. Our children loved having everyone at the table first thing in the morning and over the years we've come to enjoy starting birthdays with this routine. This year, the problem was that Tom and I were so caught up in Danny's needs that we neglected Allison's. It didn't matter that she was an adult. We had stopped a family tradition that had begun twenty- two years ago. She felt hurt and left out. We didn't have the heart to celebrate anything.

Allison let the day go by without making a fuss. A day doesn't go by when I wish we could turn back the clock of time to give Allison the attention she deserved.

We brought Dan to the hospital early in the morning for blood tests and x-rays. Tom and I were still dazed by the diagnosis and vulnerable to tears. Dan however, had a very positive attitude. He wanted to get going with the chemotherapy treatment and this was the first step. Dan shook the hospital surgeon's hand as we were beckoned into a waiting area that was also a post-operative area for children. Dr G. patiently reviewed the procedure with the three of us, always focusing on Dan's face for questions and understanding. An incision would be made near the collarbone of his left shoulder and a round rubber catheter would be placed just below the skin. After the catheter was secured, the incision would be stitched and left to heal. Then in approximately four days, chemotherapy could begin. Dr G. told Dan that he would be put to sleep for this procedure and wouldn't feel any pain until the Novocain in the area wore off. Unfortunately this "port" as the doctor called it would prevent Danny from swimming until it healed. I looked at Dan, who had a disappointed expression on his face from that news. Somehow I knew that swimming would be the last thing on Dan's mind this summer.

As Dan was prepped for surgery, Tom and I went to the hospital cafeteria for lunch. People in scrubs and uniforms, street clothes and pajamas mingled through the cafeteria choosing their lunches and seats. I wondered what their story was, how they came to be in the same place on this day. Tom and I sat with our salads and sodas at a small round table, silent, holding hands between bites. How do people go on? I wondered. How do some people come here day after day, surrounded by sick children, knowing what they will go through and still come back, eating lunch, laughing and socializing? I didn't know that soon I would understand the importance of this routine.

When we arrived back at the operating ward, Danny was prepped for surgery, drowsy and on a small bed. He knew who we were but wasn't really awake enough to want to speak. Dr. G. came in and told us the surgery would last about one hour and then Dan would be moved into a recovery area across the hall. A kind nurse with a Mickey-Mouse scrub shirt led us to the parent's waiting room. I started to cry again and wondered how I could still have so many tears in me. She put her arm around my shoulder and held a juice box in front of my face. In spite of my anxiety I felt her compassion, which I've never forgotten.

Within an hour and a half Dan was in the recovery room, groggy and sore. A large white gauze bandage covered most of his left shoulder. Dr. G. came by and told Tom and I that the operation was successful. Oh good, I thought. Now our son can go on to receive some debilitating drugs that are supposed to kill his cancer and make him well. I was not coping well through this pre-treatment plan and I knew it. I went over to Dan's bed and kissed his forehead. He looked so beautiful to me, so small and helpless. He opened his eyes, said hello and went back to sleep. His father and I kept telling him how brave he was, that the operation was over, that he could wake up as soon as he was ready. Still, he slept. Looking back, I think he probably wanted to give us a chance to get used to his port, his long periods of sleep and let us settle down before the next round of this nightmare. Then, true to his strong spirit, Dan opened his eyes, sat up, looked at Tom and stated,

"I'll have a double cheese, large fries and a chocolate shake."

We laughed, thrilled to have our son back. Tom assured Dan that we'd stop on the way home for whatever he wanted. A nurse came by and gave Dan some juice, helped him dress and wrote instructions for wound care. We left the hospital, headed for home.

Dan got his fast-food meal (although after a few bites he fell asleep with the fries hanging from his mouth). Calmness came over us as we drove home. Dan had weathered the first major step towards his wellness. Dan had a long way to go still but we decided then and there to live each day on it's own, trying not to look beyond what was happening at the time. For now, our son was safe and whole and he was coming home with us.

Elaine has been my best friend since Biology lab in sophomore year of high school. When our teacher told us to find a lab partner for the dissection unit, we immediately looked to one another. Elaine loved to pull apart bugs, worms and any other unfortunate creature we happened to be dissecting. I, on the other hand, was a decent report writer who hated touching formaldehyde-soaked specimens. It seemed only natural that we became scientific partners.

Our friendship was born in that class and continues now more than thirty years later. Honestly, Elaine and I are as different as day and night. She is outgoing, bubbly and always has a joke to tell. She is the type of person everyone invites to their party because they know that with Elaine there, people will mingle. My personality is more serious, reflective and I am prone to stepping back in a crowd. I analyze stories, talk about the latest bestseller on the New York Times Book Review and write poetry for fun. Still, the friendship works. We have watched each other marry, cried together with joy as our babies were born and helped each other pack and unpack our homes to move numerous times. Elaine is the only person I'd ever let clean and organize my kitchen; I'm the only one she'd ever tolerate making her kitchen a mess. We are godmothers to each other's children. I can't imagine my life without her. We know we'll always be there for each other. So after telling our immediate families that Dan had cancer, I called Elaine.

"He has WHAT?"

"Cancer. Non-Hodgkin's Lymphoma."

"How the Hell did he get THAT?"

"I don't know. The doctors don't know. He starts chemotherapy next Wednesday."

"Next Wednesday? Oh my God. Well listen, he's going to be fine. And you will be too. This is just a little inconvenience that he has to go through to be well."

Sure, I thought. A little inconvenience.

"What hospital is he going to?"

"The children's hospital. Seventh floor. Elaine, he's going to be in for five days each time he has treatment. How am I going to get through this with him?"

The phone was uncomfortably quiet. Then,

"Well I know. We'll celebrate life. We'll celebrate the beginning of Dan's wellness. We'll have a Chemo party!"

"A what?"

"A Chemo party. Wednesday night I'll bring a cake, some party hats, ice cream and we'll have a party for Dan in his room."

"You know you're crazy."

"See you Wednesday."

Wednesday came and it was time to begin Dan's chemo. If he was nervous he didn't let on. His bags were packed full of video games, magazines, movies and candy. He looked like a carefree teenager headed for a weeklong vacation. We rushed through breakfast to attend morning Mass and to receive a blessing from Father K. before heading to the hospital. Watching Dan receive the blessing he became my newborn wrapped tightly in my arms, the young boy mischievously molding clay on my kitchen cabinet doors, the handsome adolescent dressed in a new suit and tie, excited for his first formal school dance. I looked at the huge wooden crucifix above the main altar.

"Please heal my son," I begged. Then I joined Tom and Danny for another trip to the children's hospital.

Entering the hospital we were directed to the Hematology and Oncology unit. The waiting room was full. I don't know why I expected us to be the only family there. Maybe it never occurred to me until this time that other families were dealing with the same trauma. I met Kevin, a robust sixteen year old with short thick brown hair, who had been treated for leukemia two years before and now was in remission. He was waiting with his mother for the results of his latest blood tests, nervously pacing the hallway, afraid that the cancer had returned. There was Jamie, a sweet four year old with wisps of blond hair on her otherwise baldhead, sitting at the small wooden children's table putting a puzzle together with her sister, while an IV dripped medicine into her left arm. Other children covered the floor space watching cartoons on their parent's laps, faces drained of energy, staring at the large animated box while a volunteer offered kind words as she passed tea and coffee to adults. Really I thought, what could she say that would comfort these parents? I looked at the children younger than Dan, some barely walking. Silently I thanked God once more for giving Dan thirteen healthy years.

Finally in the late morning Dan's name was called and we were brought into the examining room. The room was cheerful with rainbow-colored fish painted randomly on the sky blue walls, spewing crystal bubbles from their mouths. I remembered a story I often read to my students about these fish and how the lessons of friendship touched my heart. I thought of Elaine, bringing the cake and hats tonight to lift everyone's spirits.

In the center of the examining room stood a huge plastic gray hippopotamus with neon pink toenails, sweeping black eyelashes and a mouth wide open where its large peach tongue held blue and white hospital gowns and small white terrycloth towels. Two electric blue plastic chairs with silver metallic legs leaned against the left wall. I guessed these chairs were for the parents while their child was being examined. In any other circumstance I would have marveled at the creativity of the room designed. Today the creativity was lost to my numb mind.

Dr. Hamilton entered the room calmly and cordially. He asked Dan how he was feeling and then listened to Dan's heart, measured his height, weighed him and examined his ears and throat. After this he began an IV of electrolyte-stabilizing liquid in Dan's left arm. He explained that when Dan's electrolytes reached a specific number (measured through blood tests) a spinal tap would be performed. After that chemotherapy would begin. Dan wouldn't be able to eat solid foods until the chemotherapy was started. So we waited. We watched television, played video games and tried to pass the time patiently. When Dan closed his eyes and slept out of boredom I rummaged through my pocketbook for my deceased mother's blue glass rosary beads that she so often had held between her fingers in a crisis, as she quietly whispered prayers of sacrifice and love. I stared at the shiny silver image hanging from the tiny cross.

"Is this how your mother felt?" I asked the image. "I'm suffocating from the pain."

I grazed my fingers over the smooth blue beads, counting each one before stopping once again at the cross. How many rosaries could I say before Dan's body was ready to start chemotherapy? My fingers grasped the cross tightly and I began to pray…

"Our Father Who Art In Heaven…"

Time dragged on until early in the evening. Finally Dan's electrolytes reached the desired number and he was ready for the spinal tap. Dr. Hamilton decided that Dan should go to his hospital room before the tap, knowing he'd be more comfortable settled in the bed that was to be his own for the next five days. As the elevator brought us to the Oncology floor, a new nervousness filled my heart. What would it be like for Dan to live here for the next five days? We entered the floor and looked onto the large floor to ceiling windows, sun rays angled onto the floor from the setting sun. The windows were decorated with colorful finger-painted drawings of flowers, dogs and horses. Next to each drawing were words of love written by the children, patients on the floor. "I love Dr. Hamilton" and "Dr. Patty is great." My heart quieted as the nurse led us to Dan's room. Dan's room was on the left of this hallway, toward the nurse's station. Entering the room I took notice of a television, leather lounge chair, two beds (one for the patient, the other for a parent). Dan had a private bathroom and a sink on the right side of the entry wall where the door opened.

Waiting in the room were Elaine, Tommy, Allison and Ryan (Jessica had gone to the beach for a few days, needing to escape the initial round of Dan's chemo). The smell of chocolate cake filled the air and colorful yellow and blue polka dotted party hats sat on the sink counter. "Get Well Soon" balloons waved gently on the chrome faucet head.

Dan hugged everyone, seeming a bit overwhelmed by the festive environment. He changed into his hospital gown and crept into bed. It had been a long day. He was tired and hungry, knowing that food was still forbidden until the spinal tap had taken place. We tried to make small talk as we waited for Dr. Hamilton. After a while, Dr. Hamilton walked into the room and acknowledged everyone. He asked Dan if he was ready to start the chemotherapy. Dan shook his head and slowly dropped it onto his pillow, closing his eyes. Dr. Hamilton drew the bed curtain as Dan's night nurse Mary

Beth infused a pain-reducing hypnotic drug into Dan's IV. Dan became increasingly tired as Dr. Hamilton eased a large needle into the base of Dan's back, withdrawing a vial of spinal fluid. When Dr. Hamilton left the room Dan remained still, his eyes shut. Again we waited. Allison and Ryan spoke about their summer jobs; Tommy spoke about his new apartment. Tom and I listened quietly, absorbed in the surroundings of the hospital room. Finally at ten o'clock Dan began his first dose of chemotherapy. He hadn't eaten anything since the morning and by now he was too tired to care. The day wasn't like any we had imagined. Tommy, Allison and Ryan, exhausted from waiting seven hours to see Dan, kissed him goodnight, promising to visit soon. Dan managed a slight smile, shaking his head. Then as he closed his eyes for the night, Tom hugged him tightly, tracing the Sign of the Cross on his forehead.

"Love you," he gently whispered to our sleeping son. "See you tomorrow after work."

I walked Tom to the elevator willing my body to remain alert. We spoke about our relief that the first chemotherapy was underway and how we'd rely on each other's strength to get through the next five days. We made a tentative schedule so that Dan would never be left alone in the hospital. We hugged each other, wishing that clinging to each other would kill the cancer. I kissed his cheek, lingering a moment on the softness that had sustained me through so many trials. As Tom walked into the elevator I held the door for an extra second, managing a tiny smile. I felt so alone.

Returning to Dan's room I noticed Elaine on the recliner next to my bed. The cake was sagging into itself, the party hats sat untouched. The balloon strings drooped into the sink. I pushed myself onto the parent bed, my head heavy on the cold wall and realized the ache in my spent body.

"So much for the Chemo party," I sighed into the darkness of the room.

"I'm not going anywhere," Elaine answered, her voice barely audible.

"I know."

I closed my eyes, exhausted and finally slept.

It was the fifth and final day of Daniel's second round of chemotherapy. He was looking at the huge IV bag drawing chemicals into his veins. One by one, each drop entered his body, killing off any roaming cancer cells. Unfortunately, the chemo was also claiming the "good cells", especially the hair cells. Dan grew impatient for this bag to be finished. An empty bag would release Dan from the hospital for another two weeks. I, on the other hand, couldn't take my eyes off Daniel's shoulders and bed pillow. There were dark, inch-long pieces of downy hair everywhere—as though an apprentice barber had grabbed his sharpest scissors and decided to try a new style on Dan. Fine brown clumps covered his pajama, his pillow and his sheets. The loss left scaly holes in his head. I tried not to appear totally focused on what I knew would be a traumatic transformation once Dan saw himself in the mirror adjacent to his bed.

"Want to play cards?" I suggested.

Playing five-card poker had become a favorite pastime of Dan's chemotherapy.

"I have to use the bathroom first," he said weakly.

Chemotherapy was taking a toll on his strength and spirit. He eased out of bed, the IV tethered to the port in his chest, chemotherapy feeding his hair's demise. Dan shut the toilet door and my heart ached as I watched the hair dropping off the bed sheets, onto the white tile floor, leading a path to the toilet like dark brown crumbs on newly fallen snow. I wanted to scoop it up and paste it back on his translucent scalp. I said nothing. When Dan returned, I pretended that everything was status quo. As Dan sat in the lounge chair next to his bed, several more clumps cascaded to the floor. Dealing the cards in silence we averted each other's eyes, attempting to concentrate on the game.

One benefit of treatment at a children's hospital is being assigned the same nurses for each admission. It's comforting to children and parents to be greeted by familiar faces, especially in cases such as Dan's, where frequent visits last a long time. So as the three o'clock shift came in we welcomed Jeannie, a veteran oncology nurse. Dan had grown very comfortable with Jeannie, who was hip, funny and into soccer.

"Hey buddy, how's it going?"

Jeannie checked Dan's IV, his chest catheter, and looked into his mouth for sores. Dan didn't answer her, not a good sign, I knew. Jeannie then very deliberately but silently shuffled up the white bed sheets, now saturated with Dan's hair tufts and left the room. Momentarily she returned, smoothed some fresh hairless sheets onto his bed and fluffed his refurbished pillow. Then looking straight at Dan, Jeannie said without trepidation,

"Time to shave that dome, Dan. When you come back in two weeks I want your head looking like Michael Jordan's."

My mouth dropped open, catching the remaining specks of fine hair drifting aimlessly around the room. Dan's sad brown eyes welled up and his chest heaved to gain control as he let out deep sighs. He wouldn't cry, especially not in front of his nurse. In two sentences Jeannie had altered Dan's confidence, at least for the time being. We continued playing cards in silence, as he tried coming to terms with the inevitable. I knew that of all the side effects chemotherapy brought, this was the one he knew would make him look like he was sick. When his hair was gone, even strangers would suspect he had cancer.

Arriving home wasn't easy for either of us. Greeted enthusiastically by his dad and sisters and brother, they tried not to focus on Dan's scalp. But it was so obvious to Dan and me that Dan's hair loss was foremost on everyone's minds. One by one they told Dan how glad they were to have him home, relaying the latest family and friend news. They offered him snacks, movies to watch, car rides to see his friends. My heart broke as we all attempted to heal the wound in his heart. Before Dan started chemotherapy, we had all imagined how we'd help him deal with hair loss. Tom and Tommy and Ryan stated they'd shave their heads in support. Allison, Jessica, and I rattled off names of famous people who chose to be bald and we offered to buy hats for Dan to wear. We all assured him the loss would be temporary and the hair would grow back before he knew it. Now, faced with the reality of the situation, all we wanted to do was help Dan get through this by skirting the issue. Finally I suggested he take a shower and get comfortable for bed.

"I guess I'll shave this first," Dan motioned to the remaining hair on his head.

That did it. In a split second his sisters were covering his neck with bath towels. His older brother charged up the electric razor for its most challenging task.

"Let me do it."

"I want a turn."

"This is sooo cool."

The hair swiftly fell. Clump by clump it floated onto the towels as Tommy mowed Dan's entire scalp. Dan sat patiently, stiffly, on the kitchen chair, too shocked to speak as he bid a silent farewell to his prized hair; too worn out from five days of chemo to care about the finality of the moment. What happened next was like a clip from a Grade B movie. His siblings turned his skull in different directions, ignoring the neck attached to it. They marveled at the crisp, clear composition, the smooth dry skin covering the pulsating veins and bony crown. They examined the perfect parallel placement of his ears and their close proximity to his bare scalp. The holes of his hair follicles were visible, appearing like ant hills mounded on a flat sidewalk. Tom and I watched, mesmerized at the audacity of our older children. Here was our beloved son, their brother, fighting for his life and they were making light of his hair loss! In the next instant, Dan was bending over, his face to his knees, as Allison smeared gobs of creamy, velvety peanut butter over the entire shaved area of his head.

"I think the dogs are going to love this," Jessica giddily reassured him.

"Don't worry Dan," Allison piped in. "The peanut butter is brand name, not some generic knockoff. The higher the cost, the more palatable it will be."

Palatable? I was horrified. Palatable for whom? Our healthy, well-fed dogs? In my naiveté thought this peanut butter-smearing orgy was intended to close the hair follicles or even out Dan's skin color! His sisters were after all, experts in self-beautification techniques using all types of foods—lemons, oatmeal, yogurt to name a few. They could close pores, smoothen dry skin and make dull hair shine by raiding the refrigerator or pantry. I thought they were about to give Dan's bald head the same benefits. Instead, Dan's head was being prepared for a canine culinary feast!

Without another word, our three hungry, feisty dogs were slurping, gobbling and drooling the peanut butter down Dan's head. They licked every last morsel and barked for more. Obligingly, Allison and Jessica scooped more peanut butter onto Dan's head, laughing hysterically at their genius. And then the strangest, most unexpected sound filled the room. It was Dan. Laughing with a resounding bellow, he urged his sisters to "get my ears and the back of my head." He lowered his head willingly for the dogs as they licked away. He held our small Maltese in his lap so it could reach his ears. Soon the whole family was doubling over at the scene-taking place.

When the jar was empty and the dogs uncomfortably full, Jessica, Allison and Tommy hugged Danny tightly and helped him get upstairs to shower off the oily residue on his head. Meanwhile, Tom took the shaver into the bathroom and shaved his already hair-challenged head. His head would remain that way until Dan's hair began to grow after his final treatment.

I sat in the kitchen, replaying the scenes in my head. Upstairs I heard Jessica speaking to Dan.

"I knew we could turn this into something positive, Dan. The dogs definitely enjoyed your head."

Tom, now hairless, came into the kitchen and I cried. Not tears of sadness (although I was sorry Dan's and Tom's hair was temporarily gone), but tears of relief and hope. Dan had conquered a major loss in cancer treatment. Gone was the devastation, the self-pity. He was ready to move on with the remaining treatments and continue his life. I knew in my heart on this evening that Dan would be a survivor; he had acquired the attitude of a survivor.

No matter how long or short his life was going to be, Dan would make the best of it. And isn't that what being a survivor is all about? Not measuring life by numbers but through experiences and attitude. Dan, I knew, was a survivor.

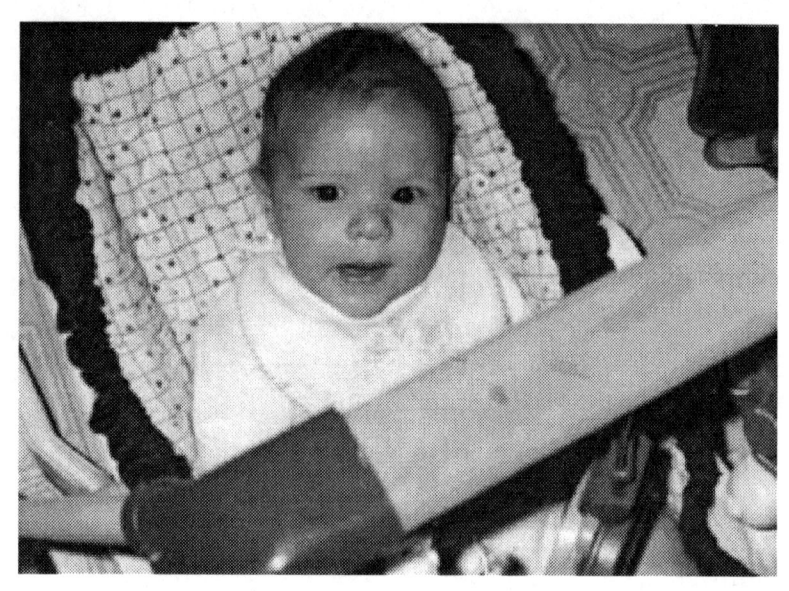

Figure 1: Dan at five months, happy and healthy

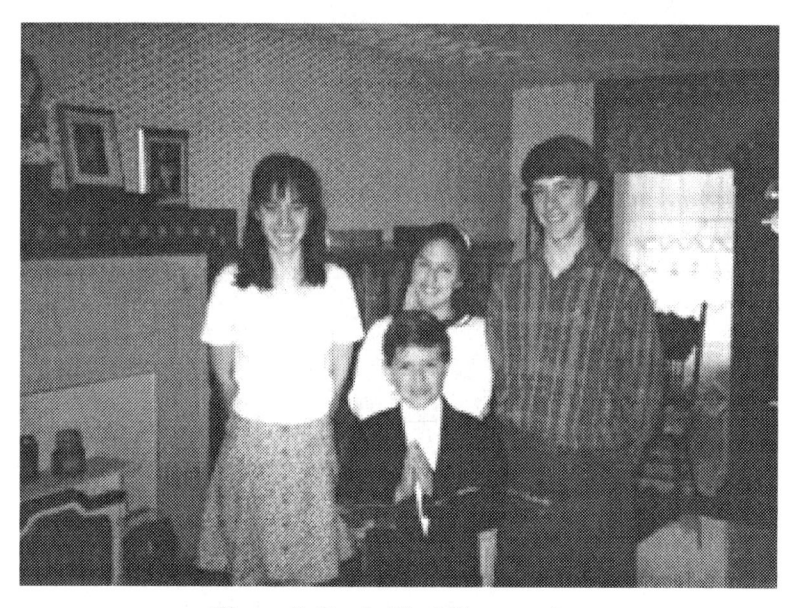

Figure 2: Dan's First Communion

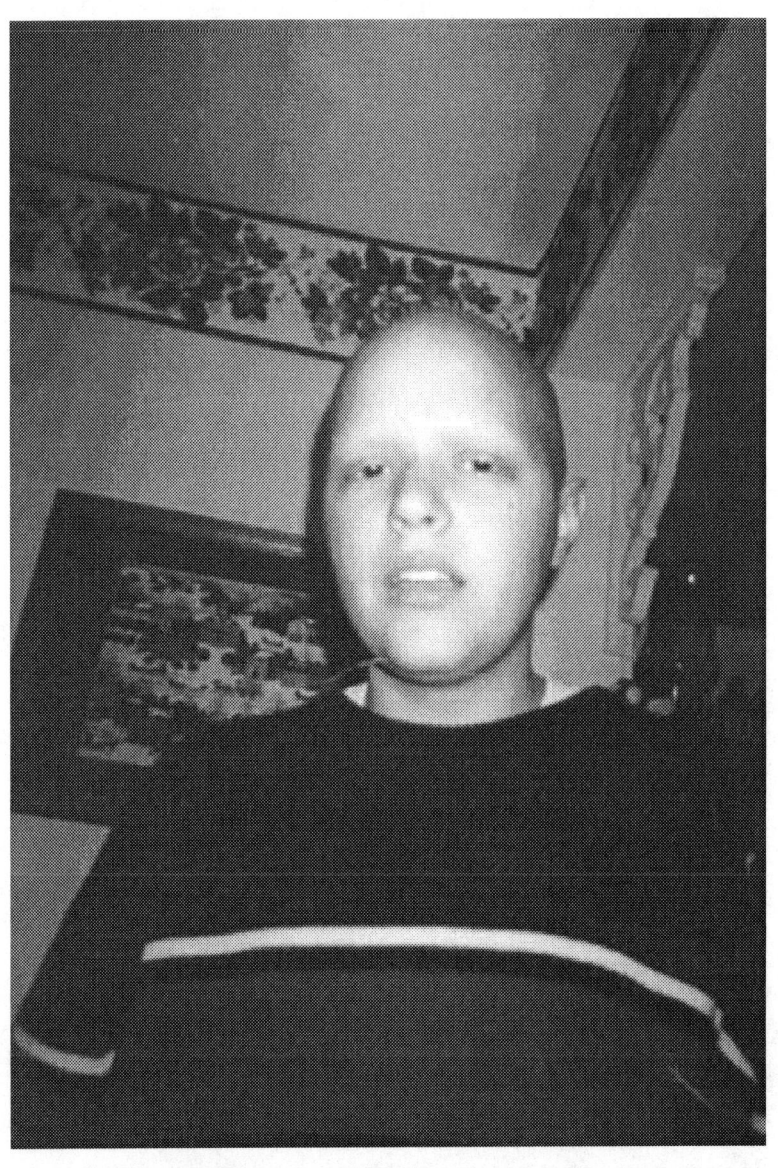

Figure 3: Dan after a long round of chemotherapy

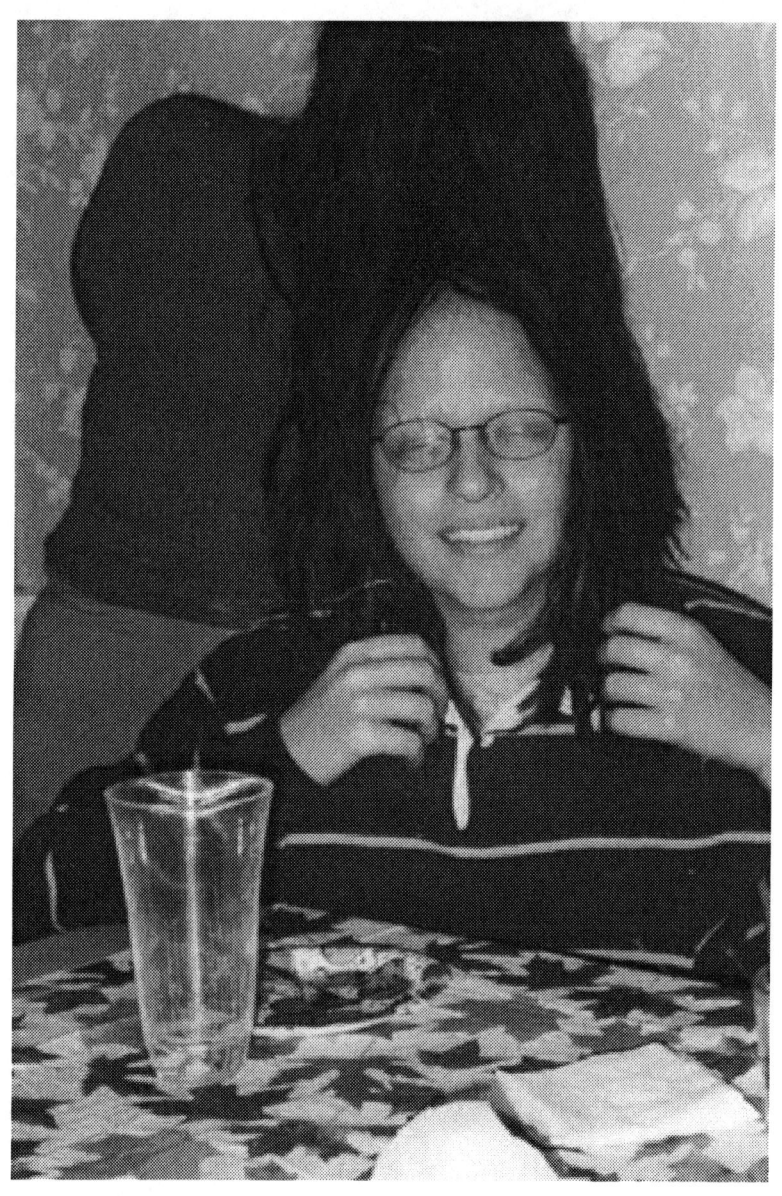

Figure 4: Using Jessica's hair when Dan had none

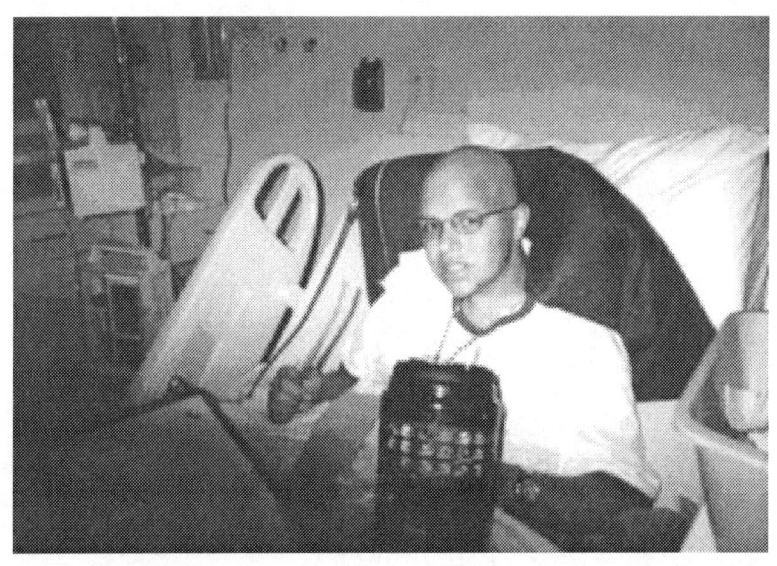

Figure 5: Chemotherapy and mouth sores take a toll

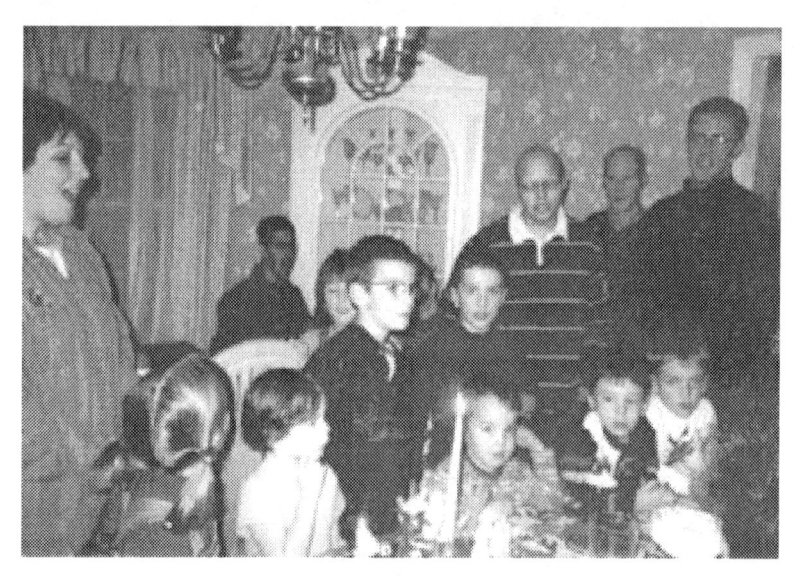

Figure 6: Thanksgiving 2001

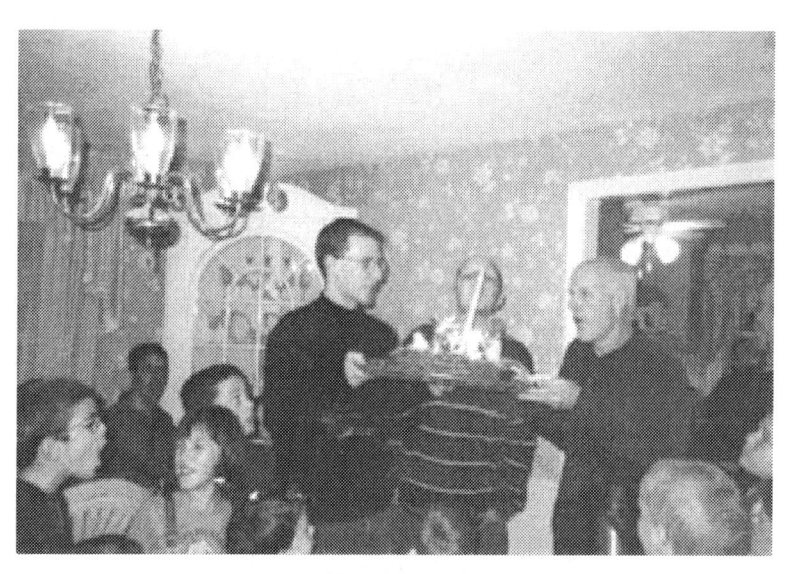

Figure 7: The No More Chemo cake

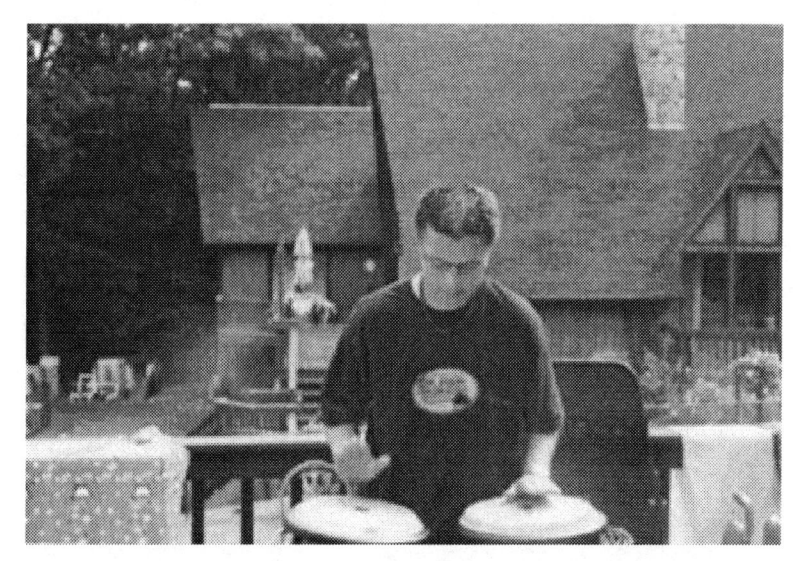

Figure 8: Dan playing the Congas, Summer 2002

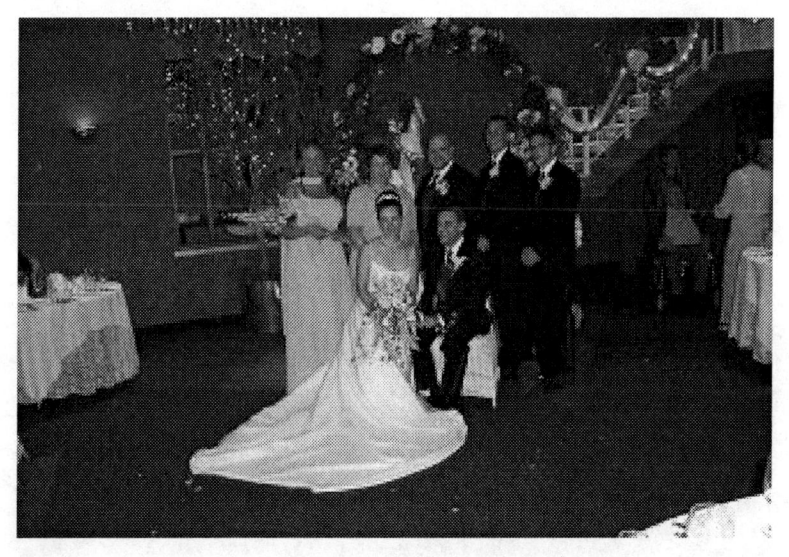

Figure 9: Allison & Ryan's wedding, 2003

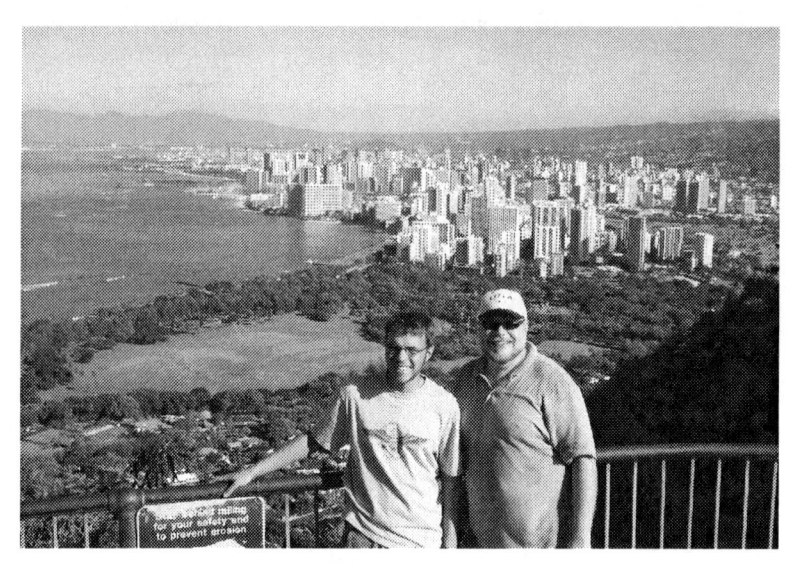

Figure 10: Dan and Dad on top of Diamond Head, Hawaii, 2004

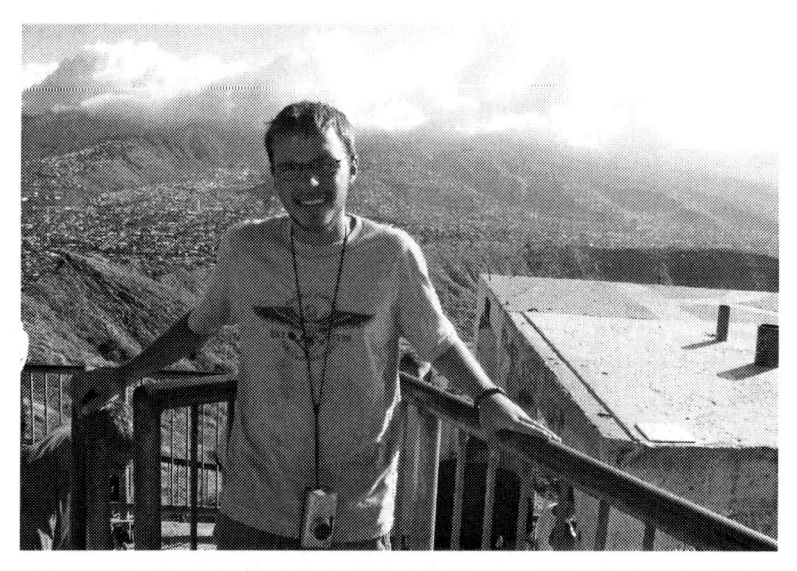

Figure 11: Dan on Top of the World; Diamond Head, August 2004

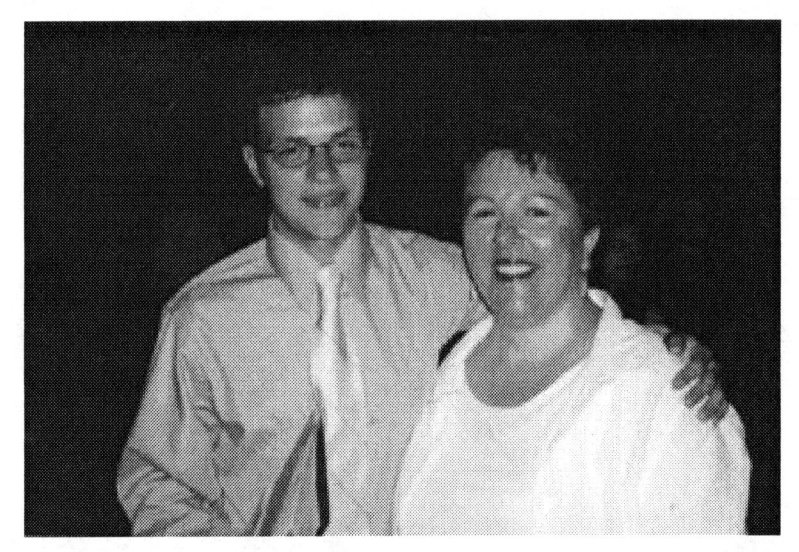

Figure 12: Dan and Mom at Senior Awards night, June , 2005

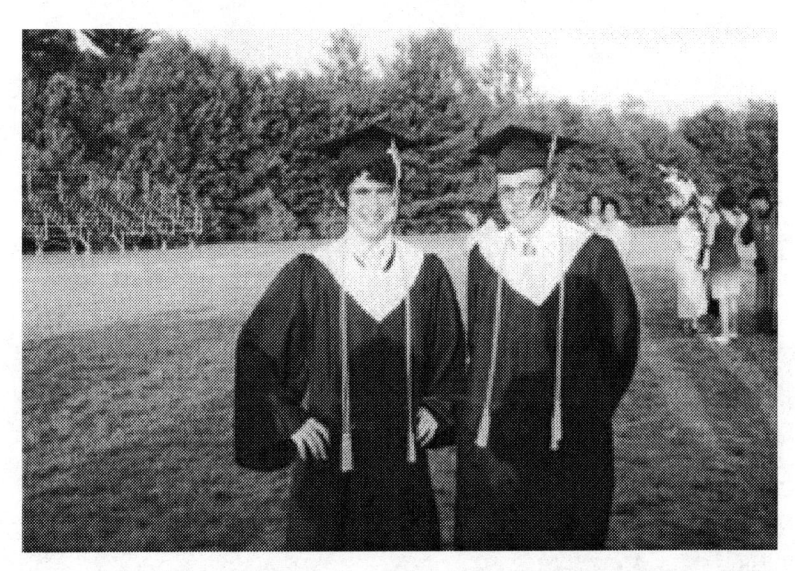

Figure13: Mike and Dan at their High School graduation, June 2005

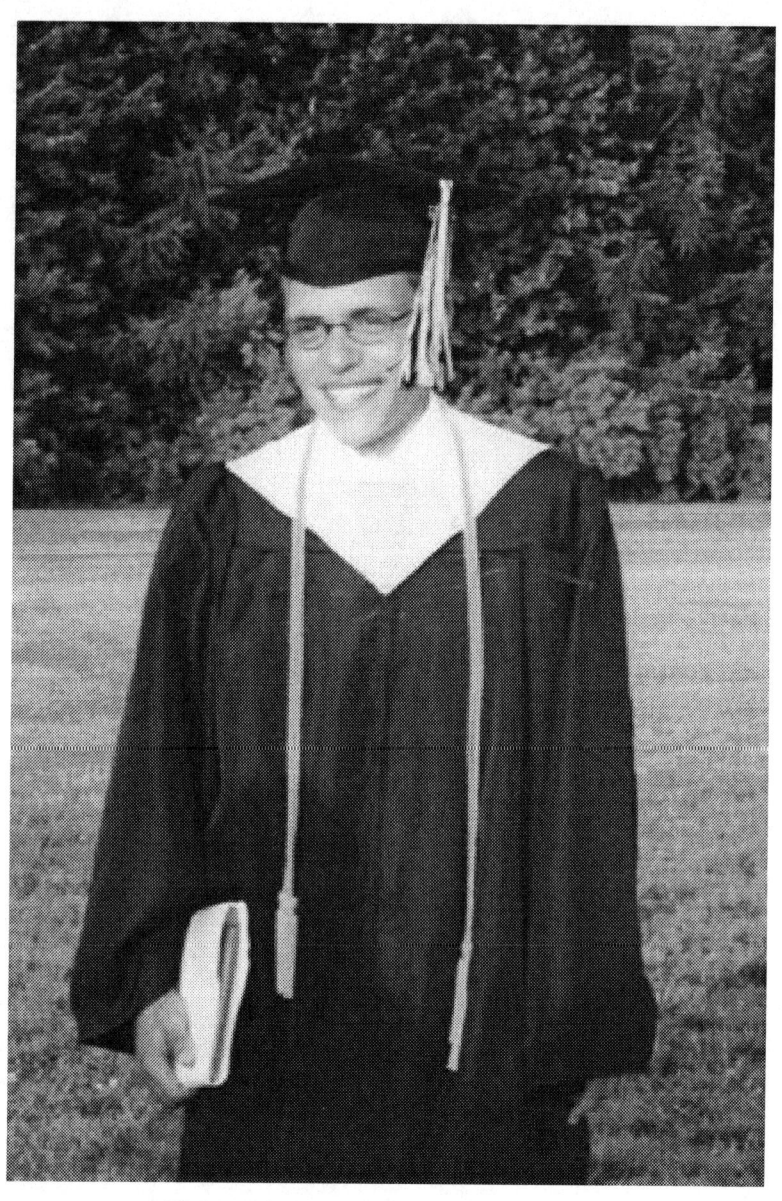

Figure 14: Dan Graduating with honors

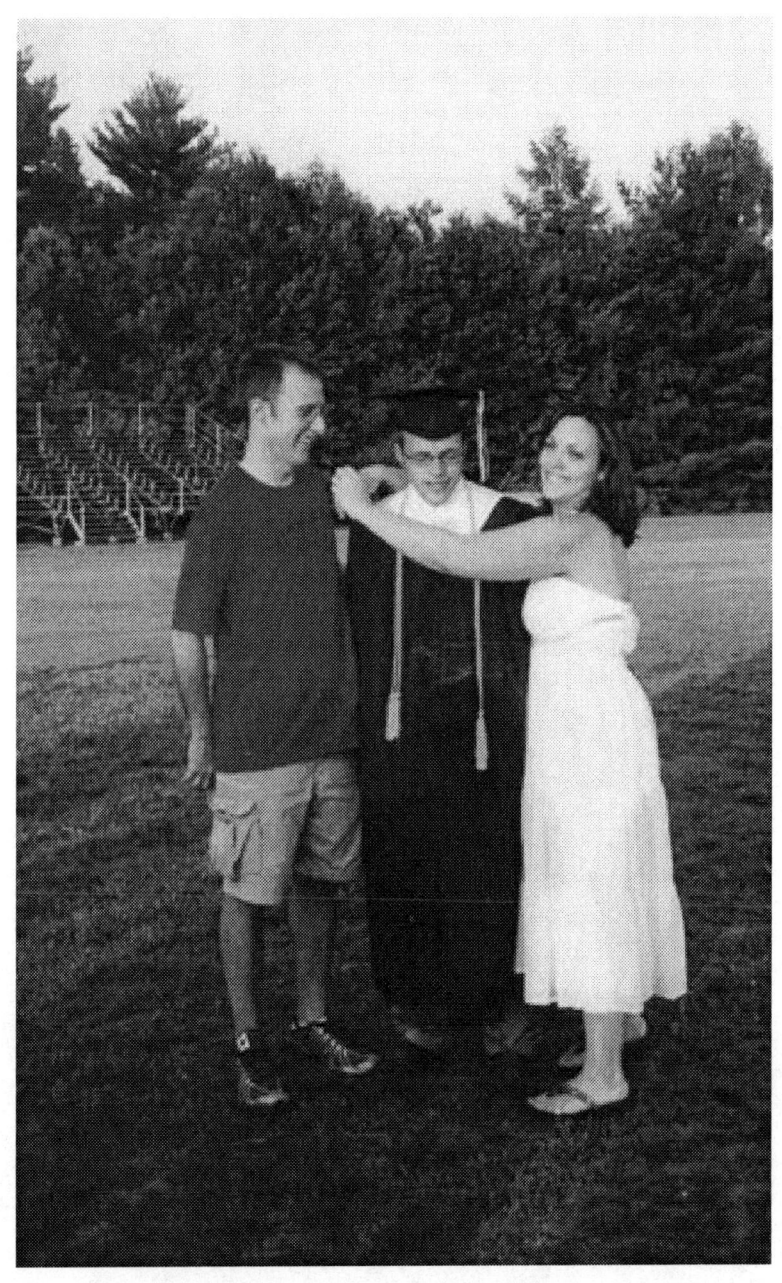

Figure 15: Tom, Dan and Jessica at Dan's Graduation

Items to Bring to the Hospital:

1. Movies
2. Clean clothes
3. Change for vending machines
4. A deck of cards
5. Magazines or books
6. A flashlight (to read magazines at night)
7. A toothbrush, deodorant, and shampoo (the hospital supplies soap and toothpaste)
8. An address book with phone numbers (It's easy to forget those numbers you're sure you'll never forget)
9. A notebook and pen (to keep track of your child's progress, medicines, and requests)
10. A religious artifact (if you choose)

Chemotherapy

I watch you in that foreign bed
Life-infusing poison dripping steadily.
"Are you here, God?" my heart screams
As the doctor checks your breath.
I look into your tired eyes
And relive your glorious birth
Of sweet-smelling milk inside my breast
Wet black hair dripping from your head.
My lips taste your salty cheek
Tears flowing on sterilized tubes.
"Only four more," I whisper
Burying my head into the crook of your arm.
Eyes closed, your hairless head nods
Breathing the sound of a gentle wind.
You take my fingers, squeezing tightly.
Sorrow branded on two souls.

Elizabeth Szewczyk
August 2001

By Dan's third round of chemotherapy, Tom and I and Dan were pretty set into a routine of admission, electrolyte balancing, spinal taps and the start of chemotherapy. We were familiar with the doctors and nurses in the infusion clinic as well as the nurses and assistants on the oncology floor. We knew their schedules and shifts, who would be around when we checked in and who would be waving goodbye as we were discharged. We had also settled into a routine within our home. Our suitcases usually sat by the side door of our family room, emptied only to wash clothes and re-pack. Dan had become partial to the oversized t-shirts that were comfortable when an IV was threaded through the armholes. He knew which shorts or boxers would protect his legs from the itch of the hospital sheets and serve as pajamas rather than having to wear those embarrassing hospital gowns. Dan had a regular rotation of movies to bring, card games to play and snacks to eat. But the one constant he still dreaded was the required spinal tap. That is, he dreaded it until the time Jessica witnessed the pre-procedural medication the nurses infused into Dan's IV—otherwise dubbed by Jessica as the "loopy" medicine.

The medicine given to Dan before the spinal tap made him relax into a euphoric twilight sleep. He could hear everything around him and was aware of the procedure but with the medicinal effect of the drug he didn't feel pain. The inhibitions he normally had dissipated.

"Dan, remember how much you love playing the trumpet?"

"Yeah," Dan would answer, getting drowsy.

"Well Dan, why don't you show Dr. Hamilton how you play?"

"OK," Dan would reply, now at Jessica's mercy due to the medication.

"Hold onto the trumpet Dan, and play *The Star Spangled Banner*."

Jessica would pass the non-existent trumpet to Dan. On cue, Dan would place his hands in a trumpet-holding position, purse his lips and start, "Bah ba bah bah bah BAAA....", his voice resending on the exact notes and finishing with the words, "Play Ball." By this time the spinal tap would be well underway and Jessica would urge Dan to play an encore of "Old McDonald Had a Farm" using his imaginary harmonica, complete with animal sounds. Dan would obligingly make cow sounds, pig sounds, rooster sounds; any sound heard on an animal farm. Dr. Hamilton would finish the "jam session" by drawing a picture of Elvis, holding a microphone, on Dan's bandage.

After this concert, Jessica would head to the hospital lobby and walk across the street to Dan's favorite eatery. She'd order a giant hamburger, mozzarella sticks, chocolate milkshakes and onion rings. Arriving back to Dan's room, Jessica would set Dan's food on a tray and then slide over to the other hospital bed. They'd eat this feast and watch movies while Dan's chemo began. Dan devoured the food, having fasted all day. He'd laugh until milk shot through his nose as Jessica replayed the spinal tap scenario. He'd ask Jessica again and again to tell him the whole story, beginning with the first injection. To a stranger passing by it appeared they were having a party. My own initial reaction to this "spinal tap spectacle" was bewilderment and embarrassment. I wasn't sure it was fair to get Dan to perform during this vulnerable time nor was I comfortable with the idea that Jessica found a spinal tap humorous. But from the first time this occurred, I watched the love and concern Jessica showed Dan. I knew she wasn't making fun of him or ridiculing him. She was finding another way to laugh at the consequences of cancer treatment. Jessica was so alarmed that Dan had to have a needle in his spine, collecting fluid to check for cancer cells, that she decided it would be much better for Dan to sing and "play" his trumpet rather than wait in silence, concentrating on the procedure.

Dan never wanted anyone but Jessica with him during the spinal tap. He'd ask his friends and family to wait in the visiting room until the chemotherapy started, was comfortable with the fact that Jessica would help him get through this procedure as no one else could. Little by little, each member of the family was finding their niche in helping Dan get through the rounds of chemotherapy. We worked together as a family in ways we never had imagined. Whether it was shaving hair, playing cards, buying hats or singing during spinal taps, we would do anything imaginable to get Dan through this ordeal.

Every year in late August my extended family gathers to celebrate the end of the summer months with a huge, old-fashioned clambake. There are more than thirty people in our family, including babies, young cousins, adult cousins, aunts and uncles and grandparents. We gather at my father's home, which borders a lake and has a sprawling backyard with a pool. Bathing suits, Frisbees and suntan lotion in tow, we arrive early in the afternoon to spend the day swimming, playing and enjoying each other's company. The lake in back of my father's home stretches for miles in length but the width enables us to gaze across to the other side as the boaters start their engines to sweep their motorboats through the clear water's crest. My father's dock holds two boats— one for pulling brave swimmers behind it in tube tires that skim the lake's foamy top as waves bounce the tires right and left with a heavy force and an eight-person paddleboat that slowly drifts from one end of the lake to the other as the occupants relax in its' open pavilion, waving to neighbors on the shore. Our clambake is a festival and a feast; we eat mounds of fish, delectable desserts and play games like softball, underwater tag and jump rope. The air smells of conversation with children and adults wanting to share vacation stories, back to school shopping expeditions and the activities that will be part of our schedules in the fall. Tom and I looked forward to this event this year especially; Dan was out of the hospital and feeling well. He was able to talk without mouth sores interfering and was strong enough to play ball and fish. But it would also be the first time since his chemotherapy began that his younger cousins saw that he was bald. Although my brothers and sisters had explained Dan's sickness to their children, nothing could prepare them to see him in person.

"What happened to your hair?" Sam asked Dan, squinting his eyes in the bright sunlight.

"The drugs used for my chemotherapy made me lose it, Sam," Dan replied, bending down, looking at his young cousin.

Soon the other cousins had gathered around Dan and Sam. Sam had asked the question that was on all their minds.

"Is that from your cancer?" John Patrick asked.

Like his other cousins, he loved Dan very much and wasn't used to seeing Dan this way. This difference was unimaginable to all of them. Dan handled the conversation with grace, speaking at their level of understanding.

"Well, it's from the drugs that help the cancer go away. The drugs kill all the bad cancer cells but they also make my hair fall out."

"I'm really sorry you have cancer, Dan," Erin said sadly.

"Thanks, Erin. It will go away soon and my hair will grow back," Dan told Erin. I could see the other children, their faces frowning.

"I'll be happy when it goes away. But your head still looks good," Morgan spoke softly for all of them.

"Thanks. I'll be happy when it goes away too."

They turned around; some held hands and went back to playing at the dock, swimming in the pool and jumping rope. I listened and thought "Wow, that's it. So simple. So direct.

So innocent." In the span of five minutes the mystery was told and solved. Everyone went back to playing their games, swimming and eating. I sighed deeply and marveled how children know what to say when they are confronted with sadness. They weren't embarrassed or afraid. They simply wanted to know why Dan's head was hairless.

The remainder of the day was relaxing and familiar. My father shared stories of his childhood; how he loved to fish with his father all day long, sitting in an aluminum rowboat, catching one or two bass for that night's supper. We laughed at the image of them pretending to be serious fishermen, quiet as mice all day long, knowing that quiet was impossible for both of them. His wife Brenda begged everyone to keep eating and my brother Jack kept yelling to everyone who came through the house,

"How about those Red Sox?" as we groaned and shook our heads, thinking this was just another baseball season as years before.

My sisters and sisters-in-law shared stories about the children; the pranks they were pulling and which adults in the family they reminded us of from long ago. Our relationship is close in spite of a large age difference. My children were teens and adults, theirs only toddlers and young scholars. But over the years I had come to know them well and I loved their presence. Along with my brothers they made me forget for just a day that the road ahead would be difficult. The sun shone brightly on the deck where we sat watching the children scream, "Marco Polo" as they dunked under the water. Dan lay on a lounge chair by the pool, in the sun and heat, determined to tan his pale head so it's color matched his arms and chest. This was just a regular family celebration. A day of togetherness, laughter, of love. I would reminisce about this day in the fall when I didn't think my heart could hold any more pain.

As the summer ended and school was about to begin, it became evident that Dan would not be starting high school in September. His treatments were taking a toll on his immune system. Often he would be readmitted to the hospital with complications the week after his chemo ended. He was susceptible to colds, infections and fevers. This left him with little energy to do much else than sleep. I knew he'd be lacking the energy to get up in the morning, put in a full day of classes and then tackle homework at night. Dan had always been a very serious student. He demanded the best he was able to produce, staying awake until late at night, rewriting reports or putting the finishing touch on projects. Feeling ill and entering a new grade would be a disastrous way for him to begin high school. In addition, soccer was the extra-curricular activity Dan loved most and he wouldn't likely play this year because of his weakening health. Tom and I decided it was time to contact the school administration for a tutor.

We broke the news to Dan shortly after his August chemotherapy. We explained our reasons for wanting him to have a tutor and shared our sorrow that he wouldn't get to start high school with his friends. I told him that I knew as a teacher the importance a tutor could make in keeping him current with the freshman curriculum. I asked him if he wanted speak with Mr. Fisher, his new principal. I thought he might like to tour the school, meet some of the teachers, and get a feel of where he'd be going when chemotherapy was finished and he had regained his strength.

The reality of the situation proved to be too discouraging for Dan. He had stoically heard the doctor review his protocol, accepted uncomfortable spinal taps, received chemotherapy that caused mouth sores and even shaved his head. But this was too much to ask a fourteen-year old boy to accept. He wanted to go to high school with his friends, to shop for back-to-school clothes and shoes. He had looked forward to picking out his classes last spring, methodically planning a four-year schedule that would allow him to take advance placement courses in his junior and senior years. This plan was now temporarily placed on hold. Most of all, he wanted to eat lunch with his friends and participate in after-school activities. Now none of this would happen as he had planned. It was the first time since his diagnosis that Dan cried in front of me. He was angry at the disease, at the injustice of cancer. I found myself telling one of my children for the second time since cancer entered our family, that nothing about this disease was fair.

I telephoned Pupil Services and explained our predicament. I was told a tutor would be hired for Dan and would be in touch with us. First though, Tom and I would need to speak with Mr. Fisher. I knew Mr. Fisher's reputation from the years my other children were in high school. I judged him to be fair and caring with his students. He had made some very positive changes since coming to our town. I was anxious to let him know Danny's plight.

Tom and I wanted to be sure Mr. Fisher saw Danny as an individual. With hundreds of students who crossed his path each day, we imagined it would be difficult for him to know each student's needs. Danny wouldn't be in school and yet he was still a member of the student community. When Danny did enter high school, we didn't want Mr. Fisher to think a new student had entered his school. So as Tom and I left the house for our meeting one summer morning, I put a picture of Danny into my pocketbook.

As we entered the cool dark hallway of the high school, Mr. Fisher, dressed in golfing shorts and a polo shirt, greeted us. I thought this was a sign that the meeting would go well—he was meeting us casually as a man who was involved in activities outside of school. I liked his casual demeanor. We shook hands and he invited us into his office—a room filled with family and school photographs, achievement plaques and books. He sat behind his desk and asked the reason for our visit.

Where do I start? I thought. I decided to tell him about Dan—as a person, a student and a son. I told him how Dan loved soccer, that his favorite food was spaghetti. I shared Dan's fondness for music and how he challenged himself repeatedly by learning new instruments. Tom spoke about Dan's academic schedule for the fall, the courses he had selected and his desire to excel. Tom stressed how important it was for Dan to be able to continue school with his class and to graduate on time. I told Mr. Fisher about Dan's bout with cancer. Then, satisfied that Mr. Fisher had a verbal biographical sketch, I took Dan's picture from my wallet and showed it to him.

"We wanted you to connect his face with the disease," I said. "We don't want you to think of Dan as the 'kid with cancer.' We want you to know him as Dan, this amazingly talented boy who unfortunately has cancer."

My throat closed, betraying my emotions. I continued.

"And we'll cooperate with you in any way we can to make sure Dan completes high school on time."

Mr. Fisher leaned towards us, his chin in the folds of his hands.

"May I keep this picture?"

I didn't know what to say. He really wanted to know Dan. He had heard everything we said and honestly cared about Dan's well being, academically and socially.

"Of course you can have his picture."

The words were barely audible. Then, with absolute resolve, Mr. Fisher assured us that Dan would graduate with his class. He could take advance placement classes during his junior and senior years. He would be allowed to enter his chosen classes as soon as his health returned.

Tom and I thanked him and stood up to leave. As we shook hands, Mr. Fisher held Dan's picture and as if speaking to Dan, said,

"Any time Dan wants to join his friends in school for lunch, or assemblies, or sports, he's most welcome. We'll let Dan call the shots on this one. Whatever he needs or wants, we'll accommodate him. And I'll keep Dan in my prayers."

Tom and I were overwhelmed by this display of kindness. We walked out of his office with a lighter step. Dan was going to have a tutor who would keep him current with his classmates until he could join them in the classroom. He'd return to school, fully participating, as he always had. Tom and I walked to the parking lot remarking what a beautiful day it was, sunny, warm and slightly breezy. It occurred to me that we hadn't stopped to enjoy the weather in a very long time. This was a great day.

~~~~~~~~~~~~~~~~~~~~~~~

After Dan's hair had fallen out and the skin on his head was completely exposed, he decided it was time to transfer his usual investment of hair products, combs and monthly cuts, to hats. Dan never wore hats too often, preferring to let his locks stand up straight with styling get. But with fall underway and winter fast approaching, Dan decided on a cool Saturday morning when he was home and feeling well, that it was time to shop for hats.

I've always tried to be the type of mother who was not possessed by name brand clothes or certain clothing stores. I unashamedly shop at bargain stores. My reasoning is if you can get what you're looking for at lower prices, you're probably better off at these stores. The items you buy will be out of style next year anyway. Besides, I love to watch the "people dynamics" while I shop. Mothers with their young children sitting squirmishly in carts, flying past underwear for new cartoon slippers, teenagers flipping through the music section, hoping the latest song they heard that morning on the radio while dressing for school hasn't sold out. And then there is the more senior group, arguing with each other over "why would you pick that laxative when the one you've been using for ten years worked so well?" It is a more informative experience than watching morning talk shows or staying awake at night for late night comedy. So, on this cool Saturday morning at the end of August, I assumed we'd be heading to one of these "sell everything" stores. I was wrong. Dan asked me to bring him to the exclusive mall thirty minutes from our home. He wanted to shop at "Hats Are Us."

"Do we have to go there, Dan?" I asked with more than a bit of hesitancy in my voice. "The stores around here have good hats."

Dan looked at me, disappointed and gloomy.

"I thought this could be like when we do 'Back to School' shopping. I thought maybe we could shop for hats and then have lunch, like we always did."

I looked at him, my son with the hairless head, half-pleading, asking for a normal day. How could I say no under the circumstances? Thirty minutes later we were at the bank, withdrawing money to cover this investment. I watched the teller counting the money to me as she finished the transaction. She looked so serious as she peered over the top of the bank window, staring at Dan's head. I wanted to tell her,

"Hey, lighten up. We're going to buy hats with this money."

Instead I remained silent, smiled as the last dollar bill crossed into my hand and walked out of the bank with Dan. We were off to the mall.

"Hats Are Us" is a very cool store for teenagers. The employees wear specialized shirts with the store logo and colorful hats to coordinate. They greet their customers at the front door, ushering them into this hat wonderland, directing them to the numerous shelves of hats.

"Are you looking for something specific?"

I looked at the salesperson incredulously. Wasn't it obvious that Dan was looking for a hat to cover his head? Fortunately, before I spoke, Dan took over the situation.

"I'm looking for some hats that I can wear with my clothes through the winter."

"Follow me," the young, stylish clerk said, trying not to focus on Dan's head.

There I was, left and forgotten in this sea of raging hormones and hats. I wasn't quite sure what to do. If I appeared to be interested in the merchandise, Dan would be mortified that he had to bring his mother to suggest one of the selections. My purpose in this expedition was to provide transportation, payment and lunch. I stood at the front of the store watching the customers come and go. There was a pair of teenage girls, their long hair grazing the curves of their waist. They were dressed stylishly in the latest red, white and blue fashion. Obviously they were serious buyers. Looking briefly around, they headed for the hats that contained only brims, which would allow their luxurious locks to wave in unison while they walked. Color was important of course. The hats, they decided, had to have different colors but the same style. I peered carefully, as they exchanged what must have been dozens of styles and colors before they decided that none suited their needs. Looking around they loudly proclaimed their tale of woe, that none of these hats would do, and oh well, they'd try one of the other upscale hat stores.

Next a group of young men entered the store. They wore t-shirts with the same orange logo that advertised another clothing store for the "under 20" crowd and faded jeans that hung loosely from their waists as the hems swept the carpeted floor. I could see by their swagger that these men were on a mission. Their goal was to find the same type of hat although not necessarily in the same color. Apparently unlike the previous merchants, they wanted to look similar so that people would know they belonged together. Between modeling and admiring their selections in the mirror, they seemed to delight in referring to one another as "Dude." Each time they took a hat off they'd say,

"Dude, my hair is totally messed up."

Then someone would pull a pocket sized black comb from his back pocket, carefully ease every loose strand of hair into place, and proceed to try on another hat. The "Dude" lingo would repeat itself for as many times as necessary until all were satisfied with the perfect hat. The choice was most often a baseball style with the rim already bent down the middle, evergreen in color with an adjustable gold buckle on the back tab. In unison they scrunched in front of the full-length mirror, meticulously combing their hair into place, preparing their heads to wear the hats. I was beginning to think that this shopping experience far surpassed the budget stores where I normally shopped, when I heard a quiet, familiar voice calling from under the knit cap turnstile.

"Pssst. Mom. Look at these."

I turned slowly, looking for any other women in the store who might remotely pass for "Mom." There were none. The caller under the knit cap section belonged to me. I eyed the merchants, making sure no one was watching and maneuvered my body under the visor rack, past the bandana rack, to the knit caps. There I found Dan, crouched tightly, his hands so full of hats he looked like he was carrying a bouquet. He had more than a dozen; knit hats, baseball hats, visor hats and ski hats.

"What do you think of these?" Dan whispered.

I paused for a minute to think. If I said they were great, that they were just perfect in color and style, he might not want any of them. On the other hand, if I said I wasn't sure about them, about their style or color, I might be locked under the knit cap section for the better part of the day while Dan selected other types of hats. I decided to be diplomatic.

"Well, what do *you* think of them?" I whispered back, my bottom half sticking out of the revolving display.

Danny reflected on the bundle in his hands.

"Well, I think these are good. I can wear them through the winter with any of my shirts and sweaters. Are there too many, Mom? Because I could put some back. I don't have to get them all."

My legs were numb and my back hurt from bending.

"I think they're just right. You should get all of them. Do you want to move towards the register? Should I give you the money now?"

"Why don't you give me the money and you can go sit outside? I'll only be a few minutes," Dan suggested.

Clearly he had thought this out carefully. Reaching through the sky blue wool hats, I passed the money like a secret agent passes a code. Then anxious to relieve my backache and anonymously disappear, I maneuvered my way through the knit cap rack, past the baseball hats and under the scarves and ski hat turnstiles. I could see the exit door. I was almost there.

"May I help you, Maam?" asked a loud masculine voice. "Are you looking for a special type of hat?"

I was caught, now surrounded by hats, teenage shoppers and employees, all staring at this middle-aged woman under the racks in the hat store.

"Lots of people your age wear our hats," he continued. "May I show you one that will cover your ears?"

I didn't know what to say. I wanted one that would cover my whole body and help me disappear, never to return to this store again. Should I tell him that the hat hunting wasn't for me but for my chemo-induced bald-headed son at the register? Or should I quickly choose a few monochromatic ski hats, try them on and pretend that I always shopped at this store? Looking around, seeing that Dan's transaction was almost complete, I shook my head slowly.

"I'm afraid you're out of my favorite style and color today," I told him with all the conviction I could muster. "Maybe when I come back in a few weeks, you'll have what I'm looking for."

With that he smiled, mumbled some words that escaped me and moved on to a group of young men and women searching for the perfect wool scarf. I slipped through the store exit feeling as though I had crossed over into the Promised Land.

"One hundred and fifty-eight dollars," Dan informed me moments later, carrying a brown, two-handled shopping bag bulging in the middle.

"And worth every penny." I answered, putting my arm around his shoulder. "Would you mind coming into the makeup store with me? There's a new eye makeup I want to try."

I was sure by now, after this unique adventure, my eyes looked as tired as I felt.

Dan shook his head. He'd wait outside the store by the fountain spurting water into a wishing pond. I nodded knowingly, shrugging my shoulders. There were just some spaces a teenage boy refused to cross.

~~~~~~~~~~~~~~~~~~~~~~~~~~

On a quiet September evening, a rare night when all of our family was at home, free from hospital comings and goings, the phone rang as we were sitting down for supper. Before Dan's diagnosis I would have let the answering machine pick up. But with test results and schedules often transferred to our home from the clinic, I answered the phone.

"Hello. Is this Mrs. Szewczyk?"

Oh no, I thought. At this hour of the day there were only two groups of people who called me "Mrs. Szewczyk." Either the call was from a school child's parent who wasn't clear about the homework assigned or it was a telemarketer. I looked at my family waiting at the dinner table, shrugged my shoulders and spoke into the phone:

"This is she," I replied, anxious to return to my family dinner. "How can I help you?"

"Well Mrs. Szewczyk, I hope I can help you," the woman sweetly replied. "This is Marie. I'm the coordinator of Children Helping Children."

My heart thumped loudly as I recalled this wonderful organization that I had read about so many times in our local newspaper. Ten years prior, a young girl Erin who lived in our town, was diagnosed with cancer. Erin was treated with chemotherapy, surgery and radiation before her cancer went into remission. During her ordeal people from the community went out of their way to cook meals for her family, send gifts and support Erin's family in any way they could. Erin decided after she had regained good health, that it was important to help other children who were suffering from a critical illness. With the support of her parents, Erin devised a low-cost carnival, complete with community gift donations and volunteers. At this one day event each year, children of all ages could be entertained by musical groups, have their faces painted by clowns, try their hand at decorating cupcakes, play Bingo and participate in many other carnival-type activities. The only charge was a small monetary donation. The proceeds from this carnival were designated each year for a sick child in the community, to be used however the child wished. Erin named this carnival "Children Helping Children." As each year passed it became more popular and by the time Danny was ill it was a renowned event in our town. Immediately when Marie identified herself I knew what the phone call was about. She went on to say that she'd heard about Danny's illness, how sorry she was that he had to go through the treatments and asked how he was doing.

"He's handling this ok. He's a strong boy," I answered, thanking her for her concern.

I went on to tell her what his prognosis was, how often he was in the hospital and that his biggest disappointment this fall was not being able to start high school with his friends.

"I think we can make Dan feel a little better," Marie said. "As you know, each year Children Helping Children puts on a carnival in October to benefit a sick child in our community."

By now, I had to sit down on the kitchen chair. My dinner was cold but it didn't matter. I couldn't believe something good was about to happen for Danny. Marie continued:

"This year, we'd like to have a double benefit, donating our proceeds to Danny and another young boy who has also been diagnosed with cancer."

Marie continued by giving me the date, the time and the place where it would be held. She ended the call by saying how much she hoped Danny would be well enough to attend that day.

I placed the phone on the receiver, stunned by this act of goodwill. Relaying the news to Dan, I calculated in my mind the treatment schedule for the October round of chemotherapy. Danny would be on his third week, which meant his chemotherapy would be finished for that round. By the third week of treatment he was usually gaining strength, able to leave home for short periods of time. Maybe he'd be able to participate in the carnival.

After a grueling September chemotherapy round, with numerous complications, including a staph infection,

October arrived. My spirits were low. Danny had never appeared weaker or less able to be with his friends and enjoy their company. It seemed that by the time we arrived home after each treatment we were heading back to the hospital because of a fever, mouth sores or a secondary infection. I put the "Children Helping Children" carnival in the back of my mind, purposely not reminding Dan about it. I thought that either Tom or I would go to the carnival to thank all of the children who were working hard for Danny. I was sure he wouldn't be well enough to even feel like making an appearance. As I traveled through our town, stopping to buy groceries or medicine, the brightly colored clown signs advertising this annual fundraiser made my heart sink. This was going to be another disappointment for Dan. I felt defeated.

Dan received his chemotherapy for October as scheduled. His treatment was the more tolerable protocol of the A/B schedule. As we looked out onto the hospital grounds from the huge window in his hospital room I noticed the leaves outside were turning vibrant shades of red, orange and yellow. They illuminated from the bright sunshine and I shared the beautiful scene with Dan. We watched the ground caretakers set large plastic pumpkins on the front lawn of the hospital. The air looked crisp and people were dressed in heavy wool sweaters. Fall had always been my favorite season. I hoped this month wouldn't be spent in a hospital room, wishing time away.

At the end of Dan's treatment he was able to return home. He was weak but not incapacitated. Only a few sores covered his mouth. I cautioned everyone at home to be especially hygienic, knowing how susceptible Dan's body was to infection. We were careful not to sneeze or cough around Dan. Lysol became my best friend. The carnival was only one weekend away. Dan stayed in the house, frustrated that I wouldn't let him go to a friend's house or have company over. But I was determined to do everything I could to get Dan well for the carnival. We ate lots of vegetables with vitamin C and drank orange juice with every meal (though I wasn't sure these would help, I decided they wouldn't hurt).

On the day of the carnival Dan woke up energetic, raring to go. He ate a larger breakfast than he had in months, downing two bowls of cereal and an enormous amount of orange juice. He dressed quickly and was on his way with his Dad to the carnival. I couldn't have asked for a better gift that day. Dan met up with many of his friends who came to show their support. He played some of the games and offered to paint faces and pumpkins. It was just the boost that Dan needed to assure him people cared and that there would be life after chemotherapy.

Later that month our family was invited to a pizza social where Dan was presented with checks from "Children Helping Children" and "Cans For Kids." Everyone who had worked to make the carnival a success attended. As I watched him accept these checks, tokens of support and best wishes, I noticed many of the past recipients smiling, clapping and laughing. They were fun-loving teenagers, having a well-deserved party after working hard for a cause they could relate to and that they believed in. I wanted Dan to be one of them, to join their hard-working circle for the benefit of another child. I wanted the time to come when Dan and our family would be able to reach beyond us, our needs and think like these smiling, clapping, laughing teenagers, "Life does go on."

During Dan's illness so many people and organizations showered Dan with gifts, lifting his spirit. He received video games from a local women's club, tickets to concerts that fulfilled wishes, even a telephone call one evening from the leader of his favorite rock band, inviting him backstage after a concert. But to me, one of the most emotional and endearing gifts he was given was a patchwork quilt made by his Great Aunt Theresa. Aunt Theresa (or Cioci as she is known from her Polish heritage) has long been a quilter in her spare time. As a member of a quilter's club, she travels throughout the eastern part of the United States, gathering materials for the patterns she makes and often donates to her church fair. When she heard that Dan was ill and would be spending the majority of his time in a hospital bed receiving chemotherapy, she decided to make Dan a quilt. No one in our family was aware of her intentions. She chose the fabric, muted shades of earth tones and lovingly placed each piece of fabric side by side, stitching them together until the quilt was large enough to cover a twin size bed. The quilt has tones of blues, reds, greens and tans and is backed with a tan and blue fabric that ties the tiny triangle pieces together. On the back is the inscription, "Made with love for Daniel J. Szewczyk, at a difficult time in his life, by his Great Aunt Theresa. October 12, 2001." Each time Dan went to the hospital the quilt went with him. We would remove the hospital blanket from his bed and replace it with the quilt. This handmade piece of love would comfort him for the next five days as Dan struggled with nausea, pain and anxiety.

Today, the quilt sits on Dan's bed at home. It isn't used for warmth or sleep. Wall collages of pictures, tickets and stuffed animals he was given during his treatments surround it as a reminder of the love he received from so many people during his diagnosis and treatment. Whenever I look at the quilt as well as the other mementos, I say a prayer of thanksgiving for the love these people have for Dan.

I've discovered that when parents meet other parents because their children are sick, sharing the same hospital floor, the same schedules of chemotherapy and the loneliness of being separated from the rest of their family, they become friends. I think this is a necessity of human nature. No one asks for this type of social gathering and I certainly would have given my own life not to be a part of it. Because I was, I will never forget two people who will always be a part of my prayers.

During Dan's first round of chemotherapy I would head into the small visiting area when Dan was asleep, just for a change of atmosphere and to read without bothering Dan. It was during this time that I met Nancy. She was a petite, bright-eyed woman, with shoulder length brown hair and a wide smile. I guessed she was in her early forties, although she appeared much younger. She had a bounce to her step as she approached me in the hall as I made my way to the reading room.

"Are you Dan's mother?" she asked me as she placed her hand on my right shoulder.

I looked at her, startled that she knew Dan. I quickly tried to place her face. No luck.

"I'm Liz Szewczyk, Dan's mom."

She went on to tell me her name and that she belonged to a prayer group in her hometown. Dan's name had come into the prayer group at their last meeting by way of our church community. Nancy went on to tell me that her daughter Kathleen had been diagnosed in early June with a rare form of brain cancer and was undergoing chemotherapy on the same rotation as Dan. The connection had been made. I asked Nancy to join me in the reading room and we talked for hours. It was the first time I had the opportunity to speak with another mother who was going through the pain I felt. Although I had spoken with mothers whose children had been treated for cancer after the news about Danny spread in our town, Nancy was the first mother who knew my pain at this very moment. Her eyes were sad as she spoke of Kathleen's life before cancer, of Kathleen's love of sports and dogs and music. She spoke about the anger she felt when she first noticed Kathleen's lack of coordination and the frustration of getting a doctor to finally consent to the tests needed for diagnosis. Nancy cried about Kathleen's pain and how she would miss school this year and probably never play in the school band again. I listened quietly and her words touch my heart. I had that same sadness and frustration for Dan. I knew Dan wouldn't be playing soccer this year or starting high school with his friends. I told her there was much more to Dan than cancer; he loved hanging out with his friends, playing soccer and he was a great joke teller. We held each other's hand as we cried for the loss of our children's innocence and carefree spirit. We nodded that our lives would never be as they had been.

Each time Danny was admitted to the hospital I would ask if Nancy and Kathleen were also on the floor. When they were I would tiptoe into Kathleen's room after Dan was settled and Nancy and I would catch up on the latest prognosis for our children. We would exchange stories that had happened since our last visit together, some hopeful and some not as fortunate and we would assure one another of our prayers. When Dan felt well he and I would wheel his IV to Kathleen's room and talk for a while about soccer and music, the latest computer software and movies. Kathleen would perk up by these visits, making her confinement to bed a bit more tolerable. I liked Nancy and Kathleen and knew that had we met under different circumstances we would have still become friends.

Late in October, Nancy met me in the hallway one morning where hospital personnel had set out juice and coffee. I noticed she had been crying. We sat together and she spoke about Kathleen's condition. It was worsening. The trip to Dana Farber had been cancelled. Kathleen wasn't responding to the chemotherapy anymore. The doctors didn't have any more answers or alternatives. Nancy knew that Kathleen was dying.

"What are you going to do?" I asked, my throat dry and quiet with heartache.

"I don't know. Kathleen asked Dr. Hamilton if she was going to die. He told her he thought she was."

Nancy buried her head in her hands and sobbed. I put my arm around her shoulder.

"You know Nancy, if it was Dan, I'd want him to know. I think children Kathleen and Dan's age need to prepare, to do things they need to do. They deserve time to say goodbye, in their own way."

We sat in the hallway, silent, hugging each other as the tears fell. My heart felt the daggers ripping it apart as we waded in pain.

In the weeks that followed Kathleen took a turn for the worse. Her pain tolerance decreased, her pain-relieving medicine increased. Nancy didn't come to the visiting room anymore. Her time was spent trying to make Kathleen comfortable and calm. I noticed the door windows to Kathleen's room had black paper taped over them, a signal for everyone to stay out unless invited. A few times I walked past the door when Dan was receiving chemo and Nancy would briefly come into the hall to ask about Dan. She didn't tell me about Kathleen's status anymore. She would pass along soda and uneaten cafeteria cookies to Dan because Kathleen didn't have much of an appetite. Then I'd ask to say hello to Kathleen. I'd peek into her room but most of the time she was sleeping. This beautiful girl was dying. Would this be Dan too, I wondered? I reflected on the words Dr. Hamilton had said when Kathleen asked if she was dying. He was right, I knew. Kathleen had a right to be able to prepare to say goodbye, to say the words she wanted to tell her mother, her family and her friends. And they needed to say goodbye to her. It was all part of the dying process and Kathleen was choosing her time to go. When the pain was too much and the drugs were ineffective, when her lovely mother could let her go, she would gently slip away. We weren't in the hospital when Kathleen died but I heard she went to heaven peacefully surrounded by everyone she loved. Although Dan and I knew Nancy and Kathleen for only a short while, we will never forget them. They were angels put in our path when we needed comfort that only those undergoing the same pain could understand.

~~~~~~~~~~~~~~~~~~~~~~~~

"I guess this shoots Halloween, doesn't it?" Dan said more like a statement than a question.

It was days before the big event and he had been admitted to the hospital with a fever. Dan hated going to the hospital with "just a small fever" but I had insisted. The fevers had become too frequent a condition that something more serious was about to take place, either in his mouth or elsewhere. Reluctantly Dan settled into his hospital room by hanging his usual Dave Mathews Band poster on the wall and turning MTV on the television. I called Tom at work, telling him we were here again and asked that he phone everyone at home. Tom told me he'd meet me at the hospital after work.

"We'll see about Halloween," I answered, not wanting to give Dan any false sense of hope.

Dan loved Halloween and all of the preparation and partying that went along with it. He had always helped me decorate our front porch with spider webs, pumpkins and our neighborhood famous "Bates Motel—No Vacancy" sign. He created unique tombstones out of cardboard, writing creative epitaphs. Dan would hang skeletons from these tombstones, admonishing others to "beware." Dan loved planning out his costume, carefully making certain that every prop adding to the costume's authenticity was bought. Each Halloween night before the doorbell started ringing, I would make a dinner of "boo burgers and fearless fries" for our family meal. Everyone looked forward to this traditional dinner.

Even at fourteen, Dan looked forward to going "trick-or-treating" with his friends, around the four streets contained within our neighborhood and then venturing out onto some main streets if his curfew wasn't up. He'd take a large pillowcase and a flashlight, combing each house for treats that normally would never appear in our kitchen. Afterwards Dan would empty his loot into a huge plastic orange pumpkin bowl and sort his favorites, leaving the remains for the others in the family to enjoy. His favorites always wound up in his bedroom, where months later I'd find wrappers under his bed, near his desk and in his pants pockets.

As the week progressed, Dan seemed more resigned to not going home for Halloween. Each day his fever shot up a few more degrees and the pallor of his skin was beginning to lighten to a sickly white. Dan's hemoglobin was getting lower every day, indicating the inevitable need for a transfusion. He didn't speak too much or move out of bed; another telltale sign that the previous round of chemotherapy was zapping his strength as well as his blood.

Along with the exhausted residents, Dr. Hamilton came by every day to monitor Dan, checking his mouth for sores and reviewing his chart. The day before Halloween, Dr. Hamilton stayed a few minutes longer.

"This place really rocks on Halloween, Dan. Everyone dresses up, the nurses, the residents, the whole staff. Dr. Robinson is always "Cruella de Ville", complete with a Dalmatian puppy. And I understand Kathleen's mom is going to paint everyone's face."

"Great," Dan said, half sarcastically, half politely.

I knew this conversation meant, "Don't get your hopes up, Dan." After Dr. Hamilton left, Dan closed his eyes and leaned back on his pillow. It was going to be another long, disappointing night.

During the night Dan tossed and turned, uncomfortable in his bed and feverish. As we watched movies around two o'clock in the morning I suggested he try to drink fluids and eat some ice pops. I wanted to slow any dehydration which was occurring from the fever and which would be another roadblock in discharging him before the weekend. Forget Halloween, I thought. Today was THE day and Dan was in no condition to go anywhere. Dan drank some soda and buzzed the nurse for Tylenol. Then he went back to sleep, never saying a word.

In the morning, Dr. Hamilton came down the hall dressed like the kind of clown who rides small cars in the circus. He wore a huge red polka-dotted tie, a curly orange wig, and enormous black shoes on his feet. I heard some of the younger children laughing as he made his way from room to room. The residents came dressed as Snow White and the Seven Dwarfs, and skipped through their rounds singing "Hi Ho." Dan wanted no part of this. He was missing Halloween and as far as he was concerned, everybody could just stop acting like this gaiety could be a substitute for trick-or-treating. The residents entered the room and Grumpy checked his chart.

"Hmm, no fever, Dan. Good sign."

Dan looked at me, his eyes weak but pleading. He knew that after a fever broke he still couldn't go home for another twenty-four hours. Unless that is, I consented. I looked at him and shook my head. Not this time.

The day passed quickly, in spite of Dan's depressed mood. Nursing assistants put a jester's hat on Dan's head and took his picture as the bells on the tip of the hat jingled. Cruella de Ville delivered bags filled with candy and small toys and Kathleen's mom painted pumpkin faces on everyone without a costume. Lunch arrived. Even the dietary team had attempted to raise Dan's spirits. An orange cupcake with a licorice black cat on top, sat on his tray. Dan took a few bites and threw the rest away. He didn't have an appetite for any food today. At four o'clock, Dan sat up and asked me again if he could go home for a few hours.

"No way," I answered. "Sorry Dan, but I don't want you to get another fever. It's raining and cold outside. Plus I think you're going to need a transfusion and platelets tonight. Your count is really low."

Dan just turned away, silent. I looked at him, lying in bed, the jester hat cocked to the left side of his head, the right side of his head hairless and pale. My mind journeyed back to every Halloween before this one, when he was healthy and able to run from door to door. I heard his laugh, his scary "booing", his deliberate counting of candy in my head, and my shoulders sank. Still, there was no way I was going to let him risk his health for a few hours. The answer was no—not this year. Dr. Cruella de Ville entered the room as if on cue:

"Hey Dan. Happy Halloween."

Dan turned his head and stated, "I want to go home. Just for a few hours. I want to go trick-or-treating."

"Ok," said Cruella. "You can have a three hour pass, starting at five o'clock. Be back in your bed at eight. We'll transfuse you then. And have fun."

She walked out of the room and I chased after her.

"Doctor, wait. I really need to speak with you about this."

She motioned over to the corner of the hallway near the visiting room. There I asked her how she could let my son, who needed blood transfusions, out of the hospital, knowing the risks of infection, of fever, of anything.

"Sometimes the emotional need outweighs the physical need," was her quiet reply.

I stood there dumbfounded. I felt helpless and afraid. By this time Tom had arrived at the hospital and as I returned to Dan's room he was helping Dan dress. Dan's nurse came by to remove his IV.

"Have a great time, Dan. If you fall and bleed, get back here immediately. And don't eat any hard candy or chips because they can cause gum bleeding. See you at eight."

Dan nodded, the first smile on his face in days.

We drove home, Dan and Tom talking about the coming events of the evening. Dan relayed the day's events to Tom and told him how this pass would be the icing on the cake. Tom spoke about what a perfect night it was for Halloween, spooky and cool. Dan probably wouldn't need a coat on top of his costume after all, Tom told him, smiling as he drove. I watched the rain drizzle on the streets, sick to my stomach. My need to protect Dan had been thwarted and I felt powerless to fight back. "What ifs?" kept entering my mind, playing havoc with my senses. We drove into the driveway and Dan bolted out of the car into the house. He called his best friend Mike, and heard all of the night's plans. Grabbing his costume, he ran upstairs to dress.

"What do you think about all this?" I asked Tom, my voice little more than a breath.

"He'll be fine, Liz. Let him go," Tom replied.

I turned around, went into the family room, buried my head into my hands and cried. Dan came downstairs dressed as the Grim Reaper (which I could not appreciate at all). He wore a long black robe that covered his head completely, a white mask that showed only slits of his eyes and mouth, and held a gray plastic sickle. I shuddered. He measured pillowcases for the largest one. With that decision made, Dan walked to the door, ready to trick-or-treat.

"We need to get back to the hospital by eight," Tom reminded him. "Have a great time."

I don't remember how I passed the next hour and a half. I'm sure I handed out candy to princesses and pirates, ghosts and goblins. I probably refilled the plastic pumpkin bowl several times and checked the jack o' lantern candle. I must have watched television in between answering the doorbell and relocating dirty dinner dishes from the sink to the dishwasher and into the kitchen cabinets. I don't remember. What I do know is that this was the longest, most heart sickening Halloween of my life and I couldn't wait for it to be over.

At seven thirty-five, Dan came bounding through the porch door, his pillowcase flowing with edible treasures. My heart quieted. Thank God he was home.

"Did you have a good time?" I asked him, trying to sound like this was an uneventful Halloween.

"Mom, it was great. All the guys went together. We covered almost the whole neighborhood and I realized it was seven fifteen. I started heading back at that time. Sorry if I'm a little late."

Dan's voice was strong and steady, unusual considering his need for a transfusion and platelets.

"You know what the best part was, Mom?" He didn't give me time to ask. "The best part was that for the first time since I was diagnosed, I felt like a normal kid."

Tears flooded my eyes. Dan continued,

"No one knew I have cancer or I'm bald or that I need blood transfusions. They couldn't see my head or my face. It was so cool. I felt like a normal kid."

I took him in my arms, hugging him, kissing his head and pasty white face, silently thanking Dr. Robinson for her insight. Sometimes the emotional does outweigh the physical.

Dan was nearing his final chemotherapy treatment. Although our entire family was anxious for his last treatment, Dan was exhausted and sick. He once again was admitted to the hospital with complications. His mouth, the effects of chemotherapy taking it's toll, was inflamed and sore. This time the sores were getting out of control.

When a person receiving chemotherapy develops mouth sores it's as though hundreds of canker sores cover the mouth. The sores make swallowing, eating, or talking difficult if not impossible. As the sores become more active the patient's fever rises. This was Dan's condition this time. I had never seen him so sick. He didn't argue about being admitted to the hospital; he didn't ask when he'd be going home. He just lay in bed, his pale head glued to the pillow, his eyes closed. Dan's fever was high and his tests indicated the need for multiple transfusions, which were impossible to give due to the fever. A morphine IV hung on a pole at the head of his bed, dripping pain relief. For the first time since July, I felt we might lose him. He didn't appear to have any fight left.

During this time I stayed by his side without leaving. I was afraid that if I left, even for a moment, he would get worse. I tried to make Dan as comfortable as possible by washing his head with a cool washcloth and placing tiny pieces of ice on his tongue. I encouraged him to sip small amounts of apple juice. He drank some juice in the early morning but by the afternoon he was refusing the ice and the juice. His fever was causing the washcloth to expel heat from his head and he became unresponsive. Dr. Hamilton came into the room as evening began:

"Hi Dan. Can you hear me, buddy? How are you feeling?"

Dan moaned a low guttural moan.

Dr Hamilton rubbed the stethoscope with his hands to warm it and listened to Dan's heart. He took Dan's pulse. I saw the seriousness in his face, the wrinkle of his brow and I knew this was different from the other times Dan had been admitted with complications. I didn't ask any questions or express concerns of my own. I thought that if I did he might tell me more than I wanted to know. Dr. Hamilton moved a gloved finger to the inside of Dan's mouth while flashing a penlight on the soft inside of Dan's cheek. I breathed deeply as the bile rose in my throat. The inside of Dan's mouth was fire engine red. Huge welts rose from the walls of his cheeks, touching each other with puss-filled knobs.

"I'll be back in a bit," the doctor said.

He patted Dan's hand and walked through the doorway to the next room.

I stroked Dan's head and whispered that he was doing a great job battling this terrible cancer. I reminded him that all of this was temporary; he would get through it and his life would return to normal. I closed the wooden door to his room, shut off the lights, and carefully tucked Cioci Theresa's handmade quilt around his body. I put my head on his chest and sang "Danny Boy", the Irish melody he loved to hear at bedtime when he was a toddler. As the song caught in my throat the second time I sang it, I noticed a tear drop slowly onto my blouse. When I looked up, Dan's eyes were closed and his face was wet. I sang the song again. And again. And again.

By early evening it was clear that Dan needed more serious intervention. His white blood cell count was virtually non-existent, leaving him susceptible to life-threatening infections. Multiple blood transfusions would have to take place within the next few hours. Dan's beautiful soft tan skin was translucent and clammy; only his cheeks contained color. They flamed crimson from the fever. His male nurse John came into the room. John gently placed the tip of a thermometer into Dan's mouth, lifted his wrist slightly to monitor his pulse, and listened with his stethoscope to Dan's heartbeat.

"He really needs a transfusion," John spoke softly. He sounded so sad. "I can't transfuse him until the fever breaks.

Keep putting the cool washcloths on his head. Can he swallow any Tylenol?"

Never had it occurred to me that Dan couldn't be helped, that his doctor and nurses wouldn't offer words of hope.

"He can't swallow anything, not even his own saliva."

"Well, we'll give him another hour. I'll leave these with you."

He handed me two small tablets of Tylenol.

"If he isn't able to swallow these within the next hour we may want to transfer him to Intensive Care."

I couldn't believe what I was hearing. My body froze, my face and ears flushed as warm tears covered my face. I knew that on this floor sending children to the ICU only occurred when the floor nurses couldn't effectively care for their patients.

John put his hand over mine.

"Try breaking the tablets into small pieces and giving him sips of water. I'll be right down the hall if you need me. If there's any change at all, push the call button."

I nodded and sat back into the chair by Dan's bed. My shoulders dropped into my chest as I tried to calm the hysteria within my heart. Jessica walked into Dan's room. Holding her hand, rubbing it gently with my fingers, I explained Dan's predicament. It was such a comfort to have her with me. She walked around the other side of Dan's bed and quietly spoke to Danny, telling him how important it was for him to take the medicine. She took the tablets from my hand and crushed them into a cup of warm water, coaxing Dan into taking a few sips. I placed another cool washcloth on Dan's head. The fever quickly turned the cloth warm. Reaching inside my pocketbook I pulled my mother's rosary beads from their pouch and pulled them carefully over Dan's head, down his shoulders. Then I called Tom at his pharmacy.

"Can you please close the store and come to the hospital? Dan's very sick."

I had never asked Tom to close the store during the entire ordeal of Dan's illness. He knew this was an emergency.

Sitting beside the phone, trying not to let my emotions upset Dan, I called Tom's mother. I told her that Dan was very ill and asked her to call Fr. Bill. I wanted Dan to receive the Sacrament of the Sick. Father Bill was the pastor at her church. He was a friend to our family and had visited Dan many times during his illness. Father Bill had experience working with families of sick children years ago at a hospital in New Haven. He would understand the crisis I was feeling.

"Mom, Dan's so sick today," I told her over the phone. "His mouth is so inflamed he can't even swallow the medicine to bring his fever down. I thought if Fr. Bill knew, maybe he would bring Dan the Sacrament."

I pushed the phone dial and called Allison and Tommy, asking them to come to the hospital too. Jessica was still holding Dan's hand, her head in the palm of her other hand. She pulled her lips tightly and shook her head at me. Dan still hadn't taken any Tylenol.

"I'm going to get a quick drink of water, ok?" I asked her.

"Sure, Mom. I'll stay with him for a while," she whispered.

I walked out into the hallway; bursts of cool air from doors swinging open and closed hitting my face. My eyes opened wider. The claustrophobic feeling of sitting in Dan's room all day left me. I gulped cold water from the fountain, clearing my mind of morbid thoughts. I blew breaths of air from pursed lips as I stepped back into Dan's room. Jessica was spoon-feeding the medicine to Dan. His mouth was open a crack and he swallowed tiny amounts. I changed his washcloth in silence and moved the cross on the rosary closer to his head.

"He'll be ok, Mom," Jessica smiled slightly. "He's going to be ok."

We held each other's hand and used our other to hold Dan. Tom stepped into the room. He kissed me on the forehead, wrapping his arms tightly around my shoulders. I felt myself relax as my head rubbed his chest. Then he bent down to Dan's ear, whispering words of love and encouragement. Danny opened his eyes and nodded his head—the first real movement he had made all day. Tom pulled a small metal chair to the edge of Dan's bed, sat down and patted his arm, saying, "I love you" over and over.

John entered the room, not saying a word. We all broke away from our own thoughts and waited for him to speak. After taking Dan's temperature and checking his other vital signs, a smile broke out on John's face.

"Good news. His temp is down. Not where I'd like it to be, but going in the right direction, much better than it was. I'll see how he's doing in a half hour."

As he walked out of the room I put my head on Dan's blanket and wrapped part of the rosary in my hand. I prayed for strength. It was a humbling time of faith for me. I thanked God for trusting me to be Dan's mother and asked Him to take Dan's pain away. As I prayed these words, Dan's heart thumped beside mine, bringing me back to memories of his infancy, when I would lay him on my chest when he wasn't sleepy or feeling well.

Father Bill stepped into Dan's room. He acknowledged us and moved straight to Dan. Speaking to Dan he assured him that God was here, watching over all of us. He put a purple stole around the back of his neck. Then opening his prayer book, he quietly read aloud the words of prayer as he anointed Dan's chest with holy oil. As Tommy and Allison arrived, terrified looks on their faces, Fr. Bill asked everyone to pray with him. We held hands and recited the "Our Father." The words, "Thy will be done" ran in my head over and over. We were living this prayer, placing complete trust that the Father would take care of all of us.

~~~~~~~~~~~~~~~~~~~~~~~~~~~~~

Dan didn't go into the ICU that night. After Fr. Bill's anointing and prayers he slept a bit; the first real sleep he'd had all day. When he woke he was able to swallow the rest of the medicine. His fever went down to a reasonable temperature for a transfusion and platelets. The color in his skin began to turn pink and he listened to us with open eyes, sometimes even smiling, as we spoke. Our son was back.

The next day Dan appeared much better. He took sips from a sixty-four ounce soda cup Tom brought to the hospital as a joke, to tease him about the amount of fluid he needed to replenish his body. Still not speaking, Dan began to write his needs on an erasable white board. He asked to watch television or listen to music with his headphones. These were great signs; Dan wanted us with him, although not too close. Tom and I didn't leave his side. I thanked God for His presence.

When I think back to this time of Dan's illness, I realize how little control we have without prayer and the support of people who love us. I believe with all my heart that a spiritual intervention took place that night.

~~~~~~~~~~~~~~~~~~~~~~~~~~~~~

In early November Dan received his final round of chemotherapy. He had completed six grueling rounds of the protocol we first learned about in July. Thanksgiving was near as was a party for Tom's parent's fiftieth wedding anniversary. I couldn't look forward to either of these events. According to past experiences, Dan's body would be reacting from the effects of his chemotherapy within the time frame of these events. I knew we would have to tell our families that in keeping with the routine of the past four months, Dan, Tom and I would probably be spending the latter part of November in the hospital.

The thought of missing the anniversary party and spending Thanksgiving at the hospital was very depressing. Relatives we saw once or twice a year would be visiting, especially Dan's cousins from Maryland, who were also some of his closest friends. Usually their visit meant a week of sleepovers, games and day trips. Tom's brother Bill was Dan's godfather and Bill's son Jacob was my godson. Jacob's brothers Joseph and Paul rounded out the foursome. These boys were inseparable when they were together. But this year would likely be different. Dan probably wouldn't be able to participate in either event.

Tom's parents were excited for their party and looking forward to all of their children and grandchildren attending. A Mass was planned. They would renew their wedding vows as their family witnessed the love that had endured for fifty years. A catered dinner would follow. I knew this was a once in a lifetime event. Next year their anniversary would be celebrated in its usual way.

Thanksgiving was the following Thursday, when my extended family always came to our house to celebrate the holiday as well as Tommy's birthday. Ever since my mother had passed away, Thanksgiving had been designated "my holiday." I loved preparing the meal, decorating the house and making my grandmother's family recipe of sausage stuffing. My young nieces and nephews would bound into the house, excited that we would be together for the whole day. Tommy's birthday was part of dessert and this year he would turn twenty years old—a milestone, no longer a teenager.

We prepared for what we thought was inevitable by telling all of our relatives to make their plans without us. Dan had always begun to run a fever about a week following his "B" course of chemotherapy and we didn't have any reason to believe this time would be different. Each "B" treatment had sent him to the hospital three weeks later. It was like clockwork. I called my sister Laura and asked her to have Thanksgiving dinner. Tom's mom assured me there would still be three places for us at their party. I washed my clothes and packed my bags, placing them near the family room door.

"Here we go again," I thought.

Dan received his chemotherapy on time and we came home from the hospital anxiously waiting for the treatment to affect his body. A few days before the anniversary party Dan's temperature started to rise. It was ninety-nine degrees; not quite high enough for him to enter the hospital but a warning that trouble was brewing. His mouth didn't have any sores in it though. I thought this was odd. He had always developed sores with the start of a fever. I expected Dan to tell me momentarily that he was uncomfortable.

The day of the anniversary party came. I woke up amazed that Dan still wasn't running a high temperature. He was still one degree short from going into the hospital. Still not convinced he wouldn't need hospitalization, Tom and I discussed the peculiarity that although Dan's temperature was higher than usual, his mouth was still free of sores. Should we risk his being exposed to relatives with colds, kissing and hugging him? How would we keep him from playing soccer with his cousins, running all over the yard, exposed to germs, dirt and pollen? We spoke about how much Dan had been though, that his treatments were finally over and how important it was for him to resume "normal living." His hair was beginning to sprout and the color in his face was returning to a light brown. I remembered Dr. Robinson's remarks on Halloween night about how important emotional health played in helping the body heal. With all of this in mind, Tom and I decided to risk it—we'd all be attending the anniversary party.

Writing this, I recall the sight of Danny, smiling, happy, present with our whole family, celebrating that joyous occasion. His grandparents had been strong supporters during Dan's treatments, never letting us lose hope during difficult times. They had brought Dan movies, his favorite foods and video games while he received chemotherapy. Dan's grandmother had even commissioned a bear made from Vermont with the words "Chemo Dan" on it. The bear's head of thick brown hair could be removed or replaced, depending on Dan's own hair at the time. It made the trip to the hospital every time Dan was admitted (and it now sits on his shelf at home, content with a full head of hair). Now here they were, with Dan, honoring their life-long commitment to each other. This was life at it's fullest, I thought.

After the Mass was celebrated we spent the day "catching up" with relatives we hadn't seen in years, laughing and joking. We toasted Tom's parents, Dan's health and each other. Tom and I actually relaxed long enough to sit down to a formal dinner—something we hadn't done in months. Dan's temperature remained stable and his mouth contained only three small sores. He was able to be with his cousins and talk about sports without having pain radiating from his mouth. As the party went on, he grew tired. Fortunately Tom's aunt and uncle lived next to the banquet facility. Dan walked over to their house with his cousins and rested for a while. At the end of the day he got into our car and came home with the family. It was a celebration we will never forget.

Thanksgiving approached a few days later and Danny still hadn't gone into the hospital. His temperature remained "high normal" and the mouth sores were holding at three. On Thanksgiving morning I called my sister and asked her to set the table for three more people. We wouldn't be going to the hospital this round.

Thanksgiving was as wonderful a day as the party the week before. Dr. Hamilton had called us the previous day with the latest results of Dan's blood tests and PET scans. Dan was cancer free and in remission. At the Thanksgiving table everyone said a prayer of thanks that Dan was healthy and able to celebrate. After dinner my sisters brought out a birthday cake for Tommy and a "No More Chemo" cake for Dan. As Danny and Tommy blew out their candles we cheered—Tommy's birthday was being joyfully celebrated and Dan's treatments were finished at last.

Two weeks after Thanksgiving Dan returned to the hospital to begin his monthly checkups. It was strange entering without my bags, without Chemo Dan, the handmade quilt or posters and games. We came through the hospital doors and for the first time since July we asked the woman at the admitting desk for a "short stay" pass. As we walked down the wide corridors I noticed fish tanks and children's paintings that I'd never realized were on the walls. When we arrived at the Oncology waiting room I poured a cup of coffee as I looked out of the seven feet floor to ceiling windows for the first time. Were the windows that high two months ago?

The nurses welcomed Dan as they walked by and asked Tom and I what had happened after his last chemotherapy treatment. They joked with us about how they had prepared his favorite examining room, had told the floor nurses he might be coming in any day and notified nurse John to reserve a video machine in Dan's name.

"Where in heaven's name were you?" they kidded.

Tom and I looked at each other. For an instant we were speechless. This was a moment we had never encountered with the hospital staff. Then we laughed with them as if they were long lost friends, finally found. We told them we had been busy with parties to attend, people to visit and lives to live. We told them that this Round, this time in our lives, was nothing less than a miracle.

Epilogue

Dan entered high school in the spring of 2002. Within a few weeks he had caught up with his studies in every class. He achieved high honors that term and each term after that. Dan played soccer through his high school years, earning a Varsity letter. In his junior year he was elected Activities Director of his class. It was that summer that the Make-A-Wish Foundation® of Connecticut contacted us. Dan and the rest of our family living at home went to Hawaii that August. I watched him surf on the northern shore of Oahu and nothing in my life made me happier. The Make-A-Wish Foundation® of Connecticut knew exactly how to enable a young man live his dream. In June 2005 Dan graduated with honors and entered college in the fall of 2005, majoring in Biochemistry. Dan continues to be healthy, living his life to its fullest. As for me, my bags are finally unpacked.